THE CARCINOID SYNDROME

To my wife and sons

The Carcinoid Syndrome

David G. Grahame-Smith MA MB BS PhD FRCP

Rhodes Professor of Clinical Pharmacology, University of Oxford,
Honorary Director Medical Research Council Clinical Pharmacology Unit,
Honorary Consultant Physician, United Oxford Hospitals,
Fellow of Corpus Christi College, Oxford.
Previously Senior Lecturer in Applied Pharmacology and Therapeutics,
University of London at St Mary's Hospital Medical School,
Honorary Consultant Physician, St Mary's Hospital, London.

WILLIAM HEINEMANN MEDICAL BOOKS LTD
LONDON

First published 1972

© David G. Grahame-Smith, 1972

ISBN 0 433 12560 8

Printed in Great Britain by
The Whitefriars Press Ltd., London and Tonbridge

Contents

Acknowledgements

I should like to express my gratitude to Professor W. S. Peart and Professor A. Neuberger for all their support over the last few years. I thank the Royal College of Physicians, London, and the Wellcome Trust for scholarships during which much of the work herein was carried out. These bodies and the Mental Health Research Fund financially supported my research. The help of my colleagues Dr J. I. S. Robertson and Dr A. R. Adamson and of the physicians and surgeons who have referred cases to me, is gratefully acknowledged.

D.G.G-S.

Preface

I came to the Carcinoid Syndrome first with the aim of unravelling some of the problems concerning the biosynthesis of serotonin, and stayed, fascinated by all the clinical and biological phenomena presented by the disease. The syndrome is bewildering, difficult and frustrating to manage but only by a knowledge of its pathology, biochemistry and pharmacology can the patients with the disease be helped. The secrets of the carcinoid syndrome are not yet all revealed but this monograph has been an exercise in trying to make a cohesive and meaningful up-to-date picture of the syndrome in terms of its clinical manifestations and the underlying abnormalities in the structure and function of the carcinoid tumour and its effects upon the patient. John Mayow said 'As a rule disease can scarcely keep pace with the itch to scribble about it'. One feels that the carcinoid syndrome will have no difficulty in keeping pace with the pen.

June 1972   David G. Grahame-Smith

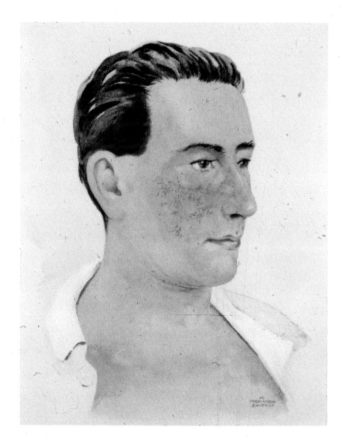

Plate 1. This is a reproduction of the picture published by Cassidy in the Proceedings of the Royal Society of Medicine (1931) showing the flushed appearance of a man with a metastatic 'adenocarcinoma' who complained of flushing, diarrhoea and had cardiac valvular lesions. This was published in 1931 before the carcinoid syndrome had been described.

CHAPTER 1

Introduction

It is necessary first to define terms and in doing so we are bound by the historical development of the subject. Oberndorfer (1907) introduced the term 'Karzenoide' ('Carcinoid') to describe a group of intestinal tumours which, although having some of the features of the more usual adenocarcinomas, were slowly growing and ran a more benign course. Gossett and Masson (1914) demonstrated that many of these tumours contained cells with granules within them which reacted with silver stains, and Masson (1928) identified the tumour cells with the Kultschitzky cells of the intestinal epithelium. Since these cells were argentaffin cells the tumours also came to be called argentaffinomas. In the period between 1952 and 1954 three groups recognized the association of certain clinical signs and symptoms in association with carcinoid tumours (Biörck, Axén and Thorson, 1952; Thorson, Biörck, Bjorkman and Waldenström, 1954; Isler and Hedinger, 1953 and Rosenbaum, Santer and Claudon, 1953) and this syndrome became variously called carcinoidosis, argentaffinosis and the carcinoid syndrome. Since then many cases of the syndrome have been described with tumours that are not argentaffin or even carcinoid in type, but the term 'Carcinoid Syndrome' has over the past few years come into general clinical usage and is here to stay as a descriptive term implying a distinctive clinical picture whatever the tumour type.

In retrospect though, it appears that isolated cases of the carcinoid syndrome had been described prior to 1952. Dr Maurice Cassidy presented a case at a meeting of the clinical section of the Royal Society of Medicine on 15 October, 1930. The patient was a 31-year-old man who had, 'Phenomenal flushing of the face, much exaggerated during emotion or during a meal. Numerous dilated venules of recent origin were present over the nose and cheeks.' Cassidy's illustration of this patient is shown in Plate 1 and his appearance is typical of one type of persistent carcinoid flushing. In addition, this patient had a mass of pelvic growth, hepatic metastases and at autopsy pulmonary stenosis. Without a doubt this was the carcinoid syndrome. Early cases of the

1

syndrome also include those reported by Millman in 1943 and Currens, Kinney and White in 1945.

However, it was with the reports already mentioned between 1952 and 1954 that the syndrome as a clinical entity gelled and in these early reports the distinctive flushing, diarrhoea, valvular lesions and bronchoconstriction were all mentioned. It seems strange that a dramatic clinical syndrome like this should have defied description until the 1950's. But what Charcot said is so true in relation to the carcinoid syndrome, 'Disease is very old and nothing about it has changed; it is we who change as we learn to recognize what was formerly imperceptible'.

In 1953 Lembeck, following up the lead afforded by Erspamer and his colleagues (see the review by Erspamer, 1954) on the presence of the pharmacologically active amine, 5-hydroxytryptamine or serotonin in the enterochromaffin cell system, isolated and characterized 5-hydroxytryptamine from a carcinoid tumour and showed that it contained a high concentration of this substance. It is ironic that this tumour was apparently not associated with the carcinoid syndrome.

The many studies of Udenfriend and his group on the mode of synthesis and metabolism of 5-hydroxytryptamine during the early 1950's quickly became of clinical relevance when forces were joined with Page and his group to show that patients with the carcinoid syndrome excreted large quantities of the 5-hydroxytryptamine metabolite, 5-hydroxyindole acetic acid, in their urine (Page, Corcoran, Udenfriend, Sjoerdsma and Weissbach, 1955). This increased excretion of 5-hydroxyindole acetic acid has remained a hallmark in the diagnosis of the syndrome even though the position of 5-hydroxytryptamine as the only active hormone secreted by the tumour has been more recently questioned, as will be discussed later. Let it suffice here to say that in addition to 5-hydroxytryptamine the roles of kallikrein, bradykinin, histamine and prostaglandins have now to be considered as agents involved in the production of the symptoms and signs of the carcinoid syndrome. In a similar expanding way and albeit that the main manifestations of the carcinoid syndrome remain those of flushing, diarrhoea, wheezing and cardiac valvular disease there is an important variability in the presentation of the syndrome which has led Sjoerdsma and Melmon (1964) to speak of the 'Carcinoid Spectrum'. This development is not just over specialization because there is no doubt that the differences in presentation of the syndrome from patient to patient reflect either a difference in the humoral products of the tumour or a variation in the individual patient's reaction to them. It is certain now that the early acceptance of 5-hydroxytryptamine as the substance solely responsible for all the manifestations of the syndrome was mistaken and that unfortunately the last line of the doggerel by Bean and Funk (1959) is probably not entirely or even partly true.

This man was addicted to moanin'.
Confusion oedema and groanin',
Intestinal rushes,
Great tricoloured blushes,
And died from too much serotonin.

To make matters more complicated, it appears that on occasions tumours producing the carcinoid syndome may also secrete ACTH, perhaps MSH and even insulin and the implications of this 'Ectopic' hormone production are most important.

Just as there has been a proliferation in the number of substances found to be produced in the syndrome, so the types of tumour found to produce the syndrome have increased. Though undoubtedly gastrointestinal carcinoids, particularly those arising in the ileum, are most commonly associated with the syndrome tumours of the bronchus, biliary tract, pancreas, and teratomas, many of which have none of the classical microscopic features of carcinoid tumours, may also produce the syndrome. However different these tumours look, the fact remains that they produce the syndrome and are functionally similar, and recent investigations of their ultrastructure are in fact beginning to reveal certain structural similarities which may relate together all the different types of tumour which can cause the carcinoid syndrome.

From the outset, therefore, it will be apparent that we shall be dealing with a disease which is heterogenous in its pathology, biochemistry, pharmacology, and clinical manifestations. The correlation of structure and function and the understanding of the basis of this heterogeneity in the carcinoid syndrome are the main themes of this text.

REFERENCES

Bean, W. B. and Funk, D. (1959). The vasculocardiac syndrome of metastatic carcinoid. *Arch. Int. Med.* **103**, 189.

Biörck, G., Axén, O. and Thorson, A. H. (1952). Unusual cyanosis in a boy with congenital pulmonary stenosis and tricuspid insufficiency. Fatal outcome after angiocardiography. *Am. Heart J.* **44**, 143.

Cassidy, M. A. (1934). Abdominal carcinomatosis associated with vasomotor disturbances. *Proc. Roy. Soc. Med.* **27**, 220.

Cassidy, M. A. (1930). Abdominal carcinomatosis with probable adrenal involvement. *Proc. Roy. Soc. Med.* **24**, 139.

Cassidy, M. A. (1931). Abdominal carcinomatosis with probable adrenal involvement. *Proc. Roy. Soc. Med.* **24**, 920.

Currens, J. H., Kinney, T. D. and White, P. D. (1945). Pulmonary stenosis with intact interventricular septum; report of eleven cases. *Am. Heart J.* **30**, 491.

Erspamer, V. (1954). Pharmacology of indolealkylamines. *Pharmacol. Rev.* **6**, 425.

Gosset, A. and Masson, P. (1914). Tumeurs endocrines de l'appendize. *Presse. Med.* **22**, 237.

Isler, P. and Hedinger, C. (1953). Metastasierendes Dünndarmcarcinoid mit schweren, vorwiegend das rechte Herz betrefferden Klappenfehlern und Pulmonalstenose— ein eigenartiger Symptomenkomplex? *Schweiz. med. Wchnschr.* **83**, 4.

Lembeck, F. (1953). 5-hydroxytryptamine in a carcinoid tumour. *Nature, London,* **172**, 910.

Masson, P. (1928). Carcinoids (argentaffin-cell tumours) and nerve hyperplasia of appendicular mucosa. *Am. J. Path.* **4**, 181.

Millman, S. (1943). Tricuspid stenosis and pulmonary stenosis complicating carcinoid of the intestine with metastases to the liver. *Am. Heart J.* **25**, 391.

Oberndorfer, S. (1907). Karizinoide: Tumoren des Dünndarms. *Frankf. Zschr. Path.* **1**, 426.

Page, I. H., Corcoran, A. C., Udenfriend, S., Sjoersdma, A. and Weissbach, H. (1955). Argentaffinoma as an endocrine tumour. *Lancet.* **1**, 198.

Rosenbaum, F. F., Santer, D. G. and Claudon, D. B. (1953). Essential telangiectasia, pulmonic and tricuspid stenosis, and neoplastic liver disease. A possible new clinical syndrome. *J. Lab. & Clin. Med.* **42**, 941.

Sjoerdsma, A. and Melmon, K. L. (1964). The Carcinoid Spectrum. *Gastroenterology,* **47**, 104.

Thorson, A., Biörck, G., Bjorkman, G. and Waldenström, J. (1954). Malignant carcinoid of the small intestine with metastases to the liver, valvular disease of the right side of the heart (pulmonary stenosis and tricuspid regurgitation with septal defects), peripheral vasomotor symptoms, bronchoconstriction and an unusual type of cyanosis: a clinical and pathologic syndrome. *Am. Heart J.* **47**, 795.

CHAPTER 2

The Cell of Origin

One of the fascinating problems highlighted by the carcinoid syndrome is the nature and function of the cell from which the tumour responsible for the syndrome arises. Here are tumour cells capable of producing several different hormones, arising often in differing anatomical sites, yet the very presentation of the carcinoid syndrome and the almost invariable association with increased 5-hydroxytryptamine synthesis shows that there is some relationship between these different types of tumour.

Let us concentrate first upon the isolated granular cells in the intestinal epithelium which were first described by Nicolas in 1891, which Kultschitzky redescribed in 1897, and which still bear his name. Schmidt (1905) found these cells to give a chromaffin reaction and two years later Ciacco (1907) called them enterochromaffin cells. Masson (1914) described the ability of these cells to take up and reduce silver salts in their granules, so called argentaffinity, and suggested that these cells were the origin of carcinoid tumours. He and Berger (Masson and Berger, 1923) in fact suggested that the enterochromaffin cells might secrete some humoral substance acting locally in the bowel wall, an example of inspired thinking. Cordier (1926) also propounded this idea and in addition showed that these enterochromaffin cells had a wide species distribution.

In 1932 Hamperl enlarged on the scope of the enterochromaffin cell system. In the argentaffin method used by Masson (1914) reliance was placed upon the ability of the intracellular granules to both fix and reduce the silver salt to produce brown or black staining. Hamperl, on the other hand, allowed tissues to fix the silver and then added an external reducing agent to reveal black granules where the silver had been fixed. This method demonstrated not only the previously described argentaffin cells but also a much wider system of cells, the 'argyrophil' cells. Since then there has been much controversy about the meaning and relationship of these two staining reactions which still continues.

Erspamer and his colleagues (see the review by Erspamer, 1954) have made an extensive study of the enterochromaffin cell system in nature and have shown these cells to be present in the gastrointestinal mucosa, biliary tract and pancreas of all vertebrates studied, with the exception of certain fish. These cells are also present in invertebrate animals, witness the use of the posterior salivary glands of the octopus for the isolation and characterization of 5-hydroxytryptamine (Erspamer and Asero, 1953). The undoubted secretory properties of the cell and its presence in such a wide distribution of species suggests that its function must be a primitive but important one in the process of evolution. Erspamer (1939) came to the conclusion that argyrophil and argentaffin cells were related, the former in some cases maturing into the latter. My own interpretation of this situation is based upon the consideration of the basis of the histochemical reactions and their meaning. Some component of the granules within both these types of cells plainly fixes silver salts. Only in the argentaffin cells is the silver reduced by endogenous components of the cell and all the evidence points to 5-hydroxytryptamine. Barter and Pearse (1953) conclusively showed that 5-hydroxytryptamine fixed in gelatin gives positive histochemical reactions. More recently Pentilla and Lempinen (1968) have studied the distribution of argentaffin and argyrophil cells in the human intestine by applying a number of histochemical techniques including argyrophil and argentaffin stains, diazo-coupling, and formaldehyde-induced fluorescence. This latter technique depends upon the conversion of 5-hydroxytryptamine to 3,4-dihydronorharman derivatives which have a yellow fluorescence and which was used by Falck (1964) to map out the cellular localization of 5-hydroxytryptamine in brain. The technique is extremely sensitive and specific for the detection of this amine in tissues. Using these techniques, Pentilla and Lempinen (1968) correlated the histochemical characteristics of various parts of the intestine with the 5-hydroxytryptamine content of those parts. They found that the fluorescence method was the most suitable for demonstrating enterochromaffin cells and this correlated well with the argyrophil method. The argentaffin method was less sensitive than either the fluorescence or argyrophil methods but more sensitive than diazo-coupling. All cells which had positive fluorescence had a positive argyrophil test but not all had a positive argentaffin test. They found an extremely positive correlation between enterochromaffin cells in the intestinal mucosa and the concentration of 5-hydroxytryptamine (see Table 1).

It seems probable that although argyrophilia indicates fixation of silver by some intracellular structure it does not signify a specific functional characteristic, though it may indicate a general ability to store secretory products, for the cells of the adrenal medulla, of phaeochromocytomas of the organ of Zuckerkandle and the carotid body are also argyrophilic (Hamperl, 1952). Nevertheless, argyrophilia is

TABLE 1

The correlation between the number of enterochromaffin cells and the
5-hydroxytryptamine content of different areas of the gastrointestinal tract
(Pentilla and Lempinen, 1968)

Site	Number of enterochromaffin cells/mm^3	5-hydroxytryptamine content (µg/G tissue)
Duodenum (outlet of bile duct)	1875	6.2
Duodenum (pyloric ring)	1688	4.9
Jejunum	1166	3.3
Ileum	518	1.7
Meckel's diverticulum	700	1.8
Appendix	381	1.1

one characteristic of the enterochromaffin cell. It is of interest that if an
animal is treated with reserpine which releases 5-hydroxytryptamine
from its storage granules the argentaffinity of the gastrointestinal mucosa
is markedly lessened while the argyrophilic properties are retained
(Pletscher, 1958). All these lines of evidence lead one to agree with
Bensch *et al.* (1968) that an argyrophilic enterochromaffin cell becomes
argentaffin cell when it contains sufficient 5-hydroxytryptamine to
reduce the silver salt. It is probably a matter of local 5-hydroxytrypta-
mine concentration, and this will depend upon the balance between the
rate of synthesis, storage and release of the amine. I would doubt
whether an argyrophil cell is of necessity a precursor of an argentaffin
cell. Although it may synthesize just as much 5-hydroxytryptamine it
may release it so quickly that it never becomes argentaffin and if this is
part of its functional capacity then argentaffinity may never become one
of its properties. This does have bearing upon the histochemical
techniques used in the examination of carcinoid tumours, since
formaldehyde-induced yellow fluorescence, argyrophilia and argentaffinity would be expected to correlate with the 5-hydroxytryptamine
content of the tumour and give an idea of at least one aspect of its
function.

Williams and Sandler (1963) have partially taken this approach and
have attempted to correlate the embryological derivation of the tumour,
with its histochemical properties and functional activity (see Table 2).
This approach has also been taken by Pariente *et al.* (1967).

Their classification takes as its reference point the ileal tumour derived
from the mid-gut as being most typical because it is most common and

TABLE 2

The characteristics of carcinoid tumours derived from different embryonic divisions of the gut

	Fore-gut	Mid-gut	Hind-gut
Histological structure	Tendency to be trabecular; may differ widely from classical pattern	Characteristic	Tendency to be trabecular
Argentaffin and diazo reactions	Usually negative	Positive	Often negative
Association with the carcinoid syndrome	Frequent	Frequent	None
Tumour 5-HT content	Low	High	Not detected
Urinary 5-HIAA	High	High	Normal
5-HTP secretion	Frequent	Rare	Not detected
Metastases to bone (Usually osteoblastic) and skin	Common	Unusual	Common
Association with other endocrine secretion	Frequent	Not described	Not described

its behaviour fairly predictable. This type of tumour is frequently argentaffin, contains a high concentration of 5-hydroxytryptamine and is often associated with the syndrome. Carcinoid tumours arising in hind-gut derivatives, particularly the rectum, often do not show argentaffinity, are not associated with the syndrome and contain little or no 5-hydroxytryptamine. Carcinoids derived from the fore-gut often show negative argentaffinity, a low content of 5HT (though 5HIAA excretion may be high showing that 5-hydroxytryptamine is synthesized and either metabolized by or released from the tumour) and these tumours are often associated with the carcinoid syndrome, though the syndrome may be clinically atypical and associated with other endocrine abnormalities. Many of these features will be discussed in detail later, but this type of classification is useful in indicating several points. First, that overall carcinoid tumours are neither structurally or functionally homogeneous. Second, that by consideration of the embryonic derivation of the cell of origin the structure and function of these tumours can be partly systematised. Third, that perhaps the enterochromaffin cell system has a common parent cell type which during development differentiates structurally and functionally leading to the presence of cells in different anatomical sites which, while superficially similar, have different normal functions. Fourth, that the different histochemical reactions reflect real organised differences in function rather than being haphazard differences in the cellular concentration of 5-hydroxytryptamine.

In terms of the incidence of the carcinoid syndrome and the function of its cell of origin there is one point which puzzles me very greatly, and which I shall document later. That is, that carcinoid tumours deriving from mid-gut structures are relatively common and very frequently give argentaffin reactions (Lille and Glenner, 1960) and yet overall are in fact infrequently associated with the carcinoid syndrome even in the presence of metastases. Unfortunately there is very little data upon which one can speculate as to the reason for this discrepancy. Certainly there is a case for careful and exacting clinical study of such cases to definitely exclude the carcinoid syndrome and for biochemical and histochemical studies of such tumours. Perhaps these tumours have lost the functional activity of their parent cell during the process of carcinogenesis as do tumours of other endocrine organs. It may be that the carcinoid tumour which does produce the syndrome and is therefore functionally active is the exception rather than the rule! Summarizing then, it appears that carcinoid tumours of the gastrointestinal producing the carcinoid syndrome arise from the enterochromaffin cells of the gastrointestinal mucosa (see Plate 2) and it is also probable that tumours producing the syndrome and arising in the bronchus, pancreas and biliary tract also arise from cells in these structures belonging embryologically to the enterochromaffin cell system, though it must be admitted that the superficial microscopic appearance and histochemical reactions of this latter group would seem often to belie their origin. This conclusion may be of some importance in regard to the 'Ectopic hormone' syndrome and is further discussed in Chapter 7.

The carcinoid syndrome in association with ovarian tumours also occurs (Waldenström, 1958) and recently this association has been reviewed by Chatterjee and Heather (1966). It appears that such tumours are usually teratomas containing argentaffin cell tissue. Although it is odd that, not infrequently, functioning argentaffin cell tissue is found in these teratomas, nevertheless the cell of origin of the functioning tumour mass is clear. Moertel *et al.* (1965) described a primary tumour of the thyroid associated with the carcinoid syndrome which was probably a type of medullary thyroid carcinoma. Williams (1968) has reviewed the role of the parafollicular cell system in the thyroid from which such tumours derive. There is no doubt that the parafollicular cell system contains 5-hydroxytryptamine (Falck *et al.,* 1964) and Williams (1968) has found as much as 10 μg/g of 5-hydroxytryptamine in a medullary thyroid carcinoma. More recently the case for these tumours secreting calcitonin (Tubiana *et al.,* 1968) and prostaglandins has been made (Sandler, Karim and Williams, 1968). Although the full blown carcinoid syndrome in association with medullary thyroid carcinomas is not common it may occur and the cell of origin appears to be the parafollicular thyroid cell. Carcinoid tumours have also been described as arising from the cervix uteri (Driesdens *et al.*, 1964) and the testis (Brown, 1964; Dockerty and Scheifley, 1955; Simon *et al.*, 1954) has also been the site of the primary growth. It is indeed very difficult to unify in terms of structure and function the cells of origin of all these tumours in different sites but it is likely that such tumours spring from cells of the enterochromaffin cell system or cells closely related to them, present in many different tissues (see also Chapter 7 and Weichert, 1970).

REFERENCES

Bensch, K. G., Corrin, B., Pariente, R. and Spencer, H. (1968). Oat cell carcinoma of the lung: its origin and relationship to bronchial carcinoid. *Cancer,* **22,** 1163.

Brown, N. J. (1964). The pathology of testicular tumours. Miscellaneous tumours of mainly epithelial type. *Brit. J. Urol.* **36,** Suppl., 70.

Chatterjee, K. and Heather, J. C. (1968). Carcinoid heart disease from primary ovarian tumours. *Am. J. Med.* **45,** 643.

Ciacco, C. (1907). 'Sopra Speciali Cellule Granulose della Mucosa Intestinale.' *Arch. ital. Anat. Embriol.* **6,** 482.

Cordier, R. (1926). Recherches morpholologiques et experimentales sur la cellule chromoargentaffine de l'Epithelium intestinal des Verté brés. *Arch. Biol., Paris,* **36,** 427.

Dockerty, M. B. and Scheifley, C. H. (1955). Metastasising carcinoid. Report of an unusual case with episodic cyanosis. *Am. J. Clin. Pathol.* **25,** 770.

Driessens, J., Clay, A., Adenio, L. and Demaille, A. (1964). Tumeur cervico-utérine et syndrome biologique de carcinoidose. *Arch. Anat. Pathol. Semaine. Hop.* **12,** 200.

Erspamer, V. (1939). 'Il Sistema Enterochromaffine ed 1 Suoi Rapporti con il Sistema Insulare.' *Z. Anat. Entw. Gesch.* **109,** 586.

Erspamer, V. and Asero, B. (1952). Identification of Enteramine, the specific hormone of the enterochromaffin cell system as 5-hydroxytryptamine. *Nature, London,* **169,** 800.

Falck, B. (1964). Cellular localisation of monoamines. *Prog. Brain. Res.* **8,** 28.

Falck, B., Larson, B., von Mecklenburg, C., Rosengren, E. and Svenaeus, K. (1964). On the presence of a second specific cell system in mammalian thyroid gland. *Acta Physiol. Scand.* **62,** 491.

Hamperl, H. (1952). 'Uber argyrophile Zellen?' *Virchows Arch.* **321,** 482.

Hamperl, H. (1932). 'Was sind argentaffine Zellen?' *Virchows Arch.* **286,** 811.

Kultschitzky, N. (1897). 'Zur Frage über ben Bau des Darmkanals.' *Arch. Mikr. Anat.* **49,** 7.

Lillie, R. D. and Glenner, G. G. (1960). Histochemical reactions in carcinoid tumours of the human gastrointestinal tract. *Am. J. Path.* **36,** 623.

Masson, P. (1914). La Gland Endocrine de l'Intestin chez l'Homme. *C.R. Acad. Sci., Paris,* **158,** 59.

Masson, P. and Berger, L. (1923). 'Sur un Nouveau Mode de Sécrètion Interne: La neurocinie.' *C.R. Acad. Sci. Paris,* **176,** 1748.

Moertel, C. G., Beahrs, O. H., Woolner, L. B. and Tyce, G. M. (1965). 'Malignant carcinoid syndrome' associated with non-carcinoid tumours. *New Engl. J. Med.* **273,** 244.

Nicolas, A. (1891). Recherches sur l'Epithélium de l'Intestin Grêle. *Int. Mschr. Anat. Physiol.* **8,** 1.

Pariente, R., Even, P. and Brouet, G. (1967). Etude ultrastructurale des carcinoides bronchiques; II Discussion. *Presse Med.* **75,** 221.

Pentilla, A. and Lempinen, M. (1968). Enterochromaffin cells and 5-hydroxytryptamine in the gastrointestinal tract. *Gastroenterology,* **54,** 375.

Pletscher, A. (1958). Topographical difference of the behaviour of 5-hydroxytryptamine in the gastric mucosa after reserpine administration. In *5-hydroxytryptamine* (ed. G. P. Lewis), Symposium Publication Ltd., Pergamon Press, London.

Schmidt, J. E. (1905). 'Beiträge zur normalen und pathologischen Histologie einiger Zellarten der Schleimhaut des menschlichen Darmkanales.' *Arch. Mikr. Anat.* **66,** 12.

Simon, H. B., McDonald, J. R. and Culp, O. S. (1954). Argentaffin tumour (Carcinoid) occurring in benign cystic teratoma of testide. *J. Urol.* **72,** 892.

Tubiana, M., Milhaud, G., Coutris, G., Lacour, J., Parmentier, C. and Bok, B. Medullary carcinoma and thyrocalcitonin. *Brit. Med. J.* **4,** 87.

Waldenström, J. (1958). Clinical picture of carcinoidosis. *Gastroenterology,* **35,** 565.

Williams, E. D. (1969). Tumours, hormones and cellular differentiation. *Lancet,* **2,** 1108.

Williams, E. D. (1968). 5-hydroxyindoles and the thyroid. *Adv. Pharmacol.* **6B,** 151.

Williams, E. D. and Sandler, M. (1963). The classification of carcinoid tumours. *Lancet,* **1,** 238.

CHAPTER 3

General Pathology

A search of the literature has failed to reveal a comprehensive review of the pathological features specifically shown by carcinoid tumours associated with carcinoid syndrome. There is, however, an extensive literature describing the overall pathology of gastrointestinal carcinoid tumours and I cannot find any feature, except that of definite malignancy and metastatic spread, which distinguishes carcinoid tumours not causing the syndrome from those that do. In considering the pathology of gastrointestinal carcinoid tumours producing the carcinoid syndrome it seems safe to draw upon the experience of many authors who have studied the overall pathology of these tumours whether or not they are associated with the syndrome. To illustrate the frequency with which gastrointestinal carcinoids produce the syndrome three studies are of importance. MacDonald (1956) reviewed 418,116 surgical specimens and 16,401 autopsies; 356 gastrointestinal carcinoid tumours were found but only four cases of the syndrome. Moertel and his colleagues (1961) at the Mayo Clinic reviewed 209 cases of small intestinal carcinoid tumours and found 14 cases of the syndrome. Sanders and Axtell (1964) reviewed 2,502 reports of gastrointestinal carcinoid tumours and found 77 cases of the associated syndrome. These series thus represent an incidence of 1 to 7 cases of the syndrome to every 100 cases of gastrointestinal carcinoids.

Carcinoid tumours appear to arise anywhere in the gastrointestinal tract (except the oesophagus). Ileal tumours most commonly produce the syndrome, gastric and jejunal sometimes. I am not aware of a duodenal or rectal carcinoid producing the syndrome, though carcinoids arise in these sites. Two cases of functional carcinoid tumours in Meckel's diverticulum have been described (Lennard-Jones and Snow, 1956). Appendiceal carcinoid tumours are common but rarely produce the syndrome.

The overall incidence, in terms of anatomical site, or gastrointestinal carcinoids is given in Table 3 (Sanders and Axtell, 1964). Moertel *et al.* (1961) give the site incidence in their series of 209 cases of small intestinal carcinoid tumours (Table 4). Davis (1960) reviewed patients

12

TABLE 3

The anatomical distribution of carcinoid tumours in the gastrointestinal tract (from Sanders and Axtell, 1964)

Site	Number	% with metastases
Stomach	86	28
Duodenum	64	23
Jejunum and Ileum	841	33
Appendix	1173	2.9
Meckel's diverticulum	30	17
Caecum	40	71
Colon	28	52
Rectum	302	28
Gall Bladder	5	0
Abdominal Metastases (no primary found)	10*	10

* 8 of these patients had the carcinoid syndrome.

TABLE 4

The anatomical distribution of small intestinal carcinoid tumours (Moertel *et al.*, 1961)

Site	Number of patients
Duodenum	4
Jejunum	15
Meckel's diverticulum	5
Ileum total*	185
Upper	17
Middle	23
Lower	86
Terminal 2 ft	70

*The site in the ileum was not stated in 50 other cases.

with malignant carcinoid tumours and his incidence by site is shown in Table 5.

Examination of these distributions and others (Wilson, 1963) reveal that appendiceal carcinoids are by far the most common. Small intestinal tumours are next most common and as these are by far the most frequent in causing the syndrome their pathology is worthy of closer examination. Examination of the data of Moertel *et al.* (1961) reveals

TABLE 5

The anatomical distribution of benign and malignant carcinoid tumours
of the gastrointestinal tract (Davies, 1960)

Site	Benign	Malignant
Stomach	28	12
Duodenum	18	6
Gall Bladder	3	1
Jejunum	14	14
Ileum	101	133
Meckel's diverticulum	11	2
Appendix	233	22
Ileocaceal valve and colon	11	33
Rectum	79	18

that the carcinoid tumour is the commonest tumour of the ileum, with
the lower ileum being the area most frequently involved. The primary
lesion is firm, and its cut surface is yellowish and is usually small, most
often less than 1.5 cm in diameter and not often larger than 3.5 cm. The
primary tumour is submucosal in site and because of its small size it is
usually, but not always, asymptomatic. When symptoms are caused by
the primary growth then intussusception and surface ulceration with
gastrointestinal bleeding are events which may occur. Very occasionally
the tumour may cause chronic intestinal obstruction. It is of great
interest that carcinoid tumours of the ileum are frequently multiple (see
Plate 3). Lubasch (1888) was the first to note this and in the series
reported by Moertel *et al.* (1961a) 29% of tumours had a multicentric
origin. This figure is much greater than that for any other gastrointestinal
neoplasm. Moertel and his colleagues also point out that associated with
carcinoid tumours is a high incidence of other malignant neoplasms and
this has been found also by Foreman (1952), Pearson and Fitzgerald
(1949) and Warren and Coyle (1951). The occurrence of other
malignancies ranges through 17%, 47%, 31% to 53% in these different
series. Moertel and his colleagues compare this high incidence with the
frequency observed in their own series of other multiple cancers, 2.3% in
surgical cases and 8.1% in autopsy cases (Moertel *et al.*, 1961b). They
speculate, not unreasonably, that if an individual develops a carcinoid
tumour he has an increased susceptibility to other forms of malignant
disease.

   The primary tumour invades first the submucosal layers into the
mucosal layer (Plate 4) and then involves the peritoneum and mesentery.
Considerable fibrotic reaction is often seen around the tumour. This is

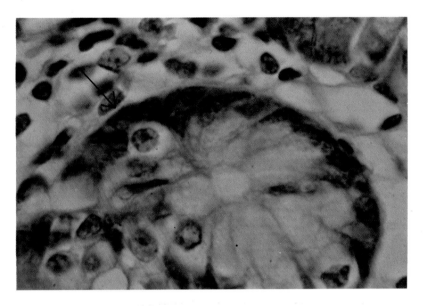

Plate 2. The enterochromaffin cell of the gastrointestinal mucosa. Section of normal ileum taken from a patient with an ileal argentaffinoma. This section shows the lower end of a crypt of Lieberkuhn and one positive diazo-staining enterochromaffin cell is marked by the arrow.

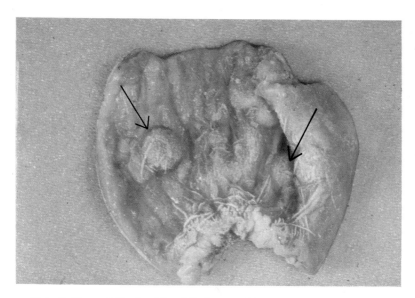

Plate 3. The multifocal origin of ileal argentaffinomas. This is a portion of an ileum removed from a patient with a malignant ileal argentaffinoma. At least five nodules were visible in this piece, two of which are marked by the arrows.

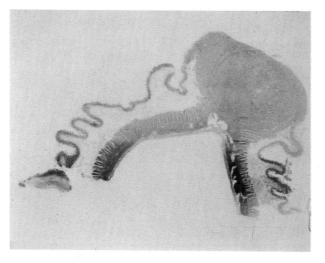

Plate 4. The local invasive properties of gastrointestinal argentaffinomas. This section shows a malignant ileal argentaffinoma locally invading the submucosal region and muscularis mucosa.

especially seen in my experience after attempted resection of the tumour. In three personal cases, after ileal resection, symptoms of intestinal obstruction have occurred and upon reopening the abdomen in the region of the resection a fibrotic mass, containing small areas of tumour, was apparent to which loops of intestine were adherent. It is likely that the tumour produces a substance which stimulates fibroblastic growth and this is discussed on page 58. Moertel also makes a point of this fibrotic reaction and found it to be responsible for 33 of 39 cases of small intestinal carcinoids in which intestinal obstruction occurred. As the tumour spreads, mesenteric lymph nodes become involved and tumour deposits may reach a large size in the mesenteric nodes, removal of which may bring some symptomatic relief in the syndrome, presumably by removal of functioning tumour tissue (Pollock, 1959). The mass of mesenteric nodes may also predispose to volvulus. Infarction of segments of the small intestine may also occur, perhaps due to obstruction of mesenteric vessels by the mass of metastatic lymph nodes, though recently Anthony and Drury (1970) have described elastic vascular sclerosis of mesenteric blood vessels associated with carcinoid tumours which may also be responsible. In relation to the production of the carcinoid syndrome other metastases are of great importance and above all, hepatic metastases appear to be almost essential for the appearance of the syndrome when the primary tumour is gastrointestinal in site, or in a site derived by the portal venous system. The reasons for this are possibly two-fold. First, and most important, the liver effectively metabolizes and therefore inactivates most of the primary tumour products. Hepatic metastases, however, drain their products into the systemic circulation via the hepatic veins, thus avoiding hepatic inactivation. Second, there may be an effect of tumour mass in that gastrointestinal tumours are usually small and the amount of humoral material they secrete is likely to be much less than that secreted by the large mass of tumour so often found in the liver. Hepatic metastases may be multiple and not too large, or they may be few and enormous (Plates 5 and 6). Just where the hepatic metastases are and their multiplicity are of importance in the consideration of hepatic surgery.

Large hepatic metastases not infrequently undergo necrosis and liquefaction producing clinical symptoms (Plate 7). Davies (1960) studied 286 patients with carcinoid tumours arising at all sites of the gastrointestinal tract and found the distribution of metastases to be that shown in Table 6.

In my own experience with ileal carcinoids associated with the syndrome, hepatic and intra-abdominal lymph node metastases are most common. Ovarian metastatic growth also frequently occurs as does involvement of the mesentery. Bony metastases are not uncommon and these are usually osteoclastic, though occasionally osteosclerotic

TABLE 6

Distribution of metastases from gastrointestinal carcinoid tumours (Davies, 1960)

Organ	Number of cases	Organ	Number of cases
Lymphatics	180	Omentum	6
Liver	137	Brain	6
Mesentery	99	Spleen	5
Peritoneum	52	Adrenal	4
Bone	11	Mediastinum	3
Lungs	10	Kidney	2
Pancreas	10	Thyroid	2
Ovary	9	Testis	1
Skin	7	Gall Bladder	1

secondaries may occur, particularly with gastric carcinoids. Williams and Sandler (1961) and Sandler (1968) point out that carcinoids arising from fore-gut and hind-gut embryonic structures more commonly give rise to bony metastases than those arising from mid-gut derivatives. However, I have seen one case of an ileal carcinoid producing the syndrome which had metastased to the vertebral column, destroying two vertebral bodies and producing paraplegia (Plate 8). Other metastases, though they in all probability do occur, have not been common in my experience.

Histological appearance

If the ileal tumour is taken as most typical (Plates 9 and 10) then the tumour is composed of small, polygonal or round cells having basophilic nuclei. The nuclei are usually central and the cytoplasm may contain lipoid vacuoles and usually granules. The cells occur in clusters, cords and sometimes show acinar and rosette formation. Between the clumps is a variable amount of stroma. The arrangement in some tumours is uniform, in others quite haphazard, varying from area to area. Mitoses are rare. The appearance, even without histochemical aids, is easily recognized in the typical tumour. Local infiltration into the submucosa and muscularis is common. Invasion locally into small blood vessels may be observed.

Histochemical reactions

Lillie and Glenner (1960) have fairly convincingly shown that when carcinoid tumours of the small intestine, caecum and appendix are promptly removed and properly preserved by formaldehyde fixation

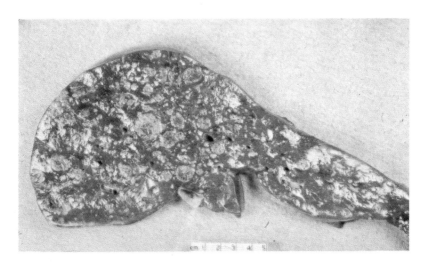

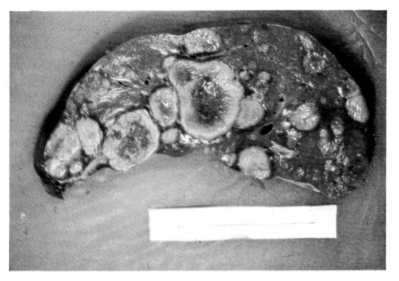

Plate 5. Multiple hepatic metastases from ileal argentaffinomas.

(a) This is a cross section of liver from a patient described in Chapter 7 who had an ileal argentaffinoma with multiple small tumour nodules in the liver as shown. This patient had the carcinoid syndrome and in addition hypoglycaemia due to hyperinsulinism.

(b) This patient also had an ileal argentaffinoma with hepatic metastases as shown, some of these were small and some were larger. The patient had the carcinoid syndrome.

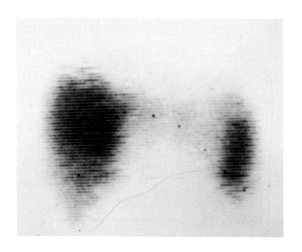

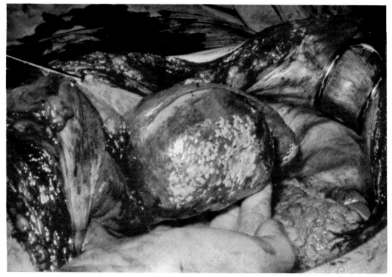

Plate 6. Represented here are:

(a) The liver scan of a patient with hepatic metastases from an ileal argentaffinoma who had the carcinoid syndrome with flushing, diarrhoea and the carcinoid heart disease. It shows almost total replacement of the left lobe of the liver by metastases.

(b) At operation this large metastasis was delivered into the wound and showed much fibrin on its surface and it did indeed replace most of the left lobe of the liver.

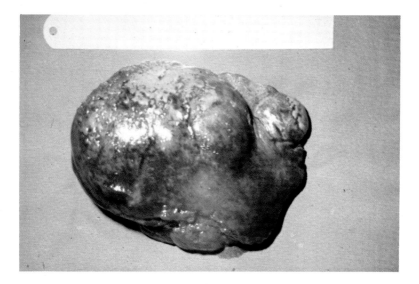

(c) The metastasis with a small edge of liver.

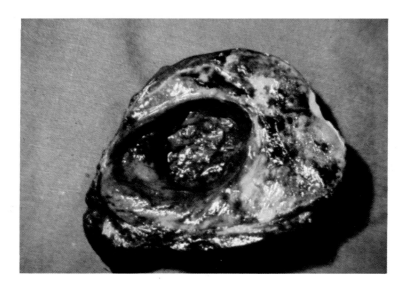

Plate 7. The large metastasis shown in Plate 6 has been cross-sectioned and shows the cavity produced by central necrosis, which can occur within these large metastatic tumours and which may be associated with intermittent worsening of symptoms.

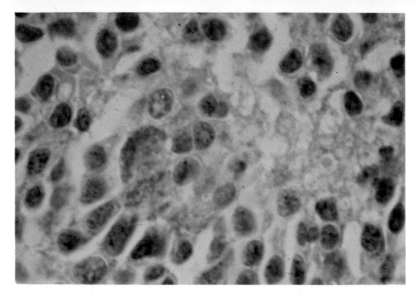

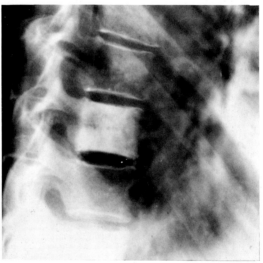

Plate 8. Vertebral metastases occurring in a patient with an ileal argentaffinoma.

(a) This patient presented, complaining only of diarrhoea. There was no complaint of spontaneous flushing. After some diagnostic difficulty the urinary 5HIAA was found to be grossly raised. Shortly after the diagnosis had been made he quite suddenly developed a paraplegia. At post mortem an ileal argentaffinoma was found which had metastasised through mesenteric lymphatics to the posterior abdominal wall and had from there invaded the vertebral column.

This figure shows diazo-staining cells of metastatic tumour tissue within the bone marrow of a vertebral body.

(b) X-ray of an osteosclerotic metastasis in a thoracic vertebra of a patient with a pancreatic tumour (an adenocarcinoma) associated with the carcinoid syndrome. Osteosclerotic deposits are most frequently seen with gastric carcinoids and other fore-gut carcinoids.

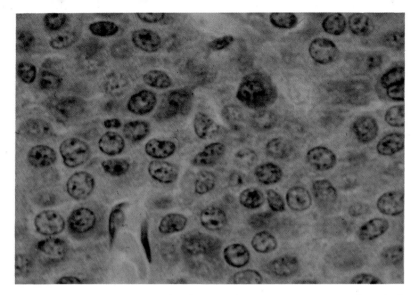

Plate 9. High power section of ileal carcinoid tumour. Diazo-reaction. Several of the cells here contain granules which show positive diazo-staining.

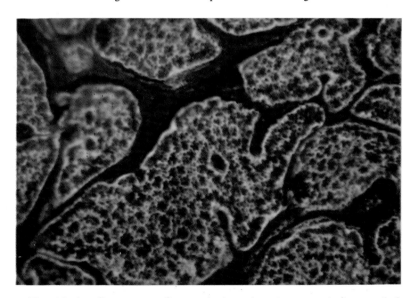

Plate 10. Autofluorescence of serotonin in an hepatic metastasis from an ileal argentaffinoma. To a section of metastatic tumour the fluorescent technique of Falck and Hillarp was applied. In ultra violet light the serotonin (5HT) fluoresces with a green colour and it can be clearly seen that serotonin is not just diffusely dispersed throughout the tumour but apparently organized around the edges of cell clusters and probably around the periphery of cells, emphasizing that even though malignant, the tumour retains functional and organized secretory properties. (I am grateful to Dr Polak, Department of Histochemistry, Hammersmith Hospital, for this section).

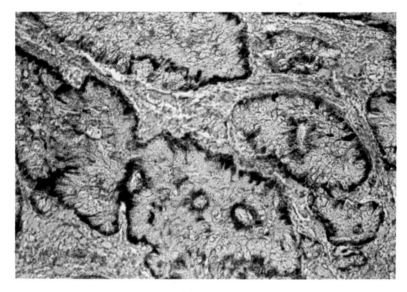

Plate 11. Section of hepatic metastasis from ileal argentaffinoma stained to reveal polypeptides by the lead-haematoxylin method. This section shows a concentration of staining material towards the edges of clusters of tumour cells and again the clumps of tumour cells show an organized secretory pattern. Such a staining reaction is characteristic of the APUD series of cells described by Professor A. G. E. Pearse and I am grateful to Dr Polak, Histochemistry Department, Hammersmith Hospital, for this section.

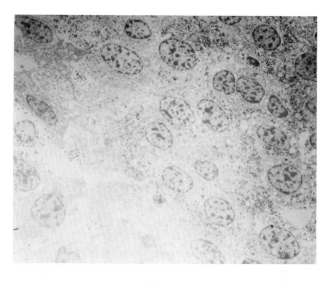

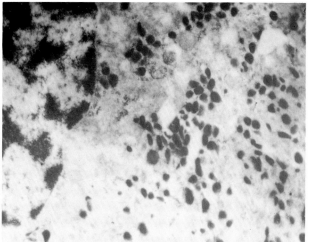

Plate 12. (a) Electron micrograph of section of hepatic metastasis from ileal argentaffinoma. This section shows the argentaffin cells with their large nuclei with granules dispersed in their cytoplasm, which are the granules to which serotonin is bound. In many of the cells these granules appear to be situated toward the periphery of the cell.

(b) High power electron micrograph from the section shown in (a). This shows the population of granules which are extremely pleomorphic, differing in both size and shape. They are, however, all very electron dense. Their difference in size and shape may account for the fact that on density gradient centrifugation there is often widespread dispersal of these granules throughout the density gradient.

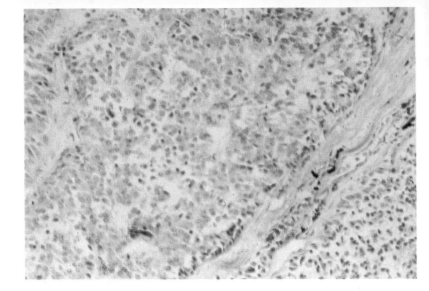

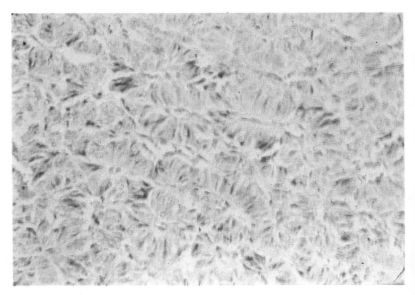

Plate 13. The pleomorphism of tumours producing the carcinoid syndrome.

(a) Section of primary tumour in the lung of a patient presenting with severe facial flushing of type 3 (see page 44). This type of flushing is typical of bronchial carcinoids. This patient also complained of severe diarrhoea. The section shows a polygonal cell carcinoma but could not be definitely classified as a carcinoid tumour nor as an oat-cell carcinoma of the bronchus. This tumour contained an excess of serotonin and the patient excreted an abnormal amount of 5HIAA in the urine.

(b) This is a section from a pancreatic tumour (Peart *et al.*, 1964) which shows a pancreatic adenocarcinoma. This tumour in no way resembled the more usual type of argentaffinoma. There was no argentaffinity or positive diazo-staining, the tumour however, did contain 5-hydroxytryptophan and 5-hydroxytryptamine in abnormally large amounts.

nearly all can be demonstrated to contain granules within their cells which show an argentaffin reaction. The same tumours also show azo-coupling and these authors advise argentaffin and azo-coupling reactions in the histological diagnosis of carcinoid tumours. Gastric and rectal carcinoids are usually negative in these reactions. Pearse (1953) also suggests that diazo reactions may be more reliable in diagnosis. Delay in fixation may result in loss in the histochemical features of argentaffin tumours and the argentaffinity varies remarkably from clump to clump of tumour cells and within any one clump as well, indicating perhaps variable biochemical function or variable capacities of cells to store 5-hydroxytryptamine. It would be of great interest to study the fluorescence characteristics of carcinoid tumours, which one would predict would be almost invariably positive in all those cases producing an excess of 5-hydroxytryptamine (see Plate 11). These histochemical reactions have been discussed in the consideration of the cell of origin and the same arguments apply here.

Recently, in co-operation with Professor A. G. E. Pearse and Dr Pollack of the Royal Postgraduate Medical School, London, I have had the opportunity to study some of the histochemical, microfluorescent and electron microscopic appearances of hepatic metastases from a carcinoid tumour of the ileum, removed at operation. Plate 12 shows the appearances found.

Appendiceal Carcinoid Tumours

The position as regards appendiceal carcinoids requires careful consideration. Although malignant appendiceal carcinoids can produce the carcinoid syndrome, nevertheless the association is rare. In their review of the literature, Moertel and his colleagues found only four cases of the carcinoid syndrome in the literature associated with tumours at this site, all having metastases. Yet the appendix is the commonest site of the carcinoid tumour, the incidence in appendices removed at operation being 0.03% to 0.5% in series of 5000 cases or more. In autopsy cases the incidence varies from 0.009% to 0.17%. In fact the appendiceal carcinoid tumour is the commonest tumour occurring in the young adult population.

Moertel and his colleagues point out that the appendiceal carcinoid tumour is potentially malignant and even without distant metastases the occurrence of invasion of the muscularis, lymphatic invasion, and invasion of the peritoneal surface is alarmingly high. Five of their 144 had ileal carcinoid tumours as well and 13% of their patients had histologically confirmed primary tumours elsewhere. They advise simple appendicectomy for patients with appendiceal carcinoid tumours in which there is no grossly recognizable evidence of metastatic spread. If lymphatic permeation is present then Right Hemicolectomy is advised, and if the tumour is 2 cm or more in diameter then similar aggressive surgery is advised.

Overall, however, the incidence of distant metastases with appendiceal carcinoids is small. Reviewing 1140 reported cases of appendiceal carcinoids and 33 cases of their own, Sanders and Axtell (1964) found distant metastases present in 2.9%. They found none in their own cases. Most appendiceal carcinoids are found either as incidental findings during intra-abdominal exploration for other reasons or in appendices removed because of appendicitis. The low incidence of metastatic spread and the removal of appendiceal carcinoids because of 'Obstructive' appendicitis perhaps accounts for their rare association with the carcinoid syndrome, but one wonders whether these can be the only reasons.

Gastric Carcinoid Tumours

Askanazy in 1923 described the first two cases of gastric carcinoid tumours. From then until 1961 Christodoulopoulos and Klotz (1961) found reports of 77 cases of gastric carcinoid tumours and added two of their own. Amongst these 79 cases there were five cases of the carcinoid syndrome (Sandler and Snow, 1958; Fein and Knudtson, 1956; Sauer *et al.*, 1958; Pochaczeosky and Sherman, 1959; Christodoulopoulos and Klotz, 1961). This incidence of 6.3% of the carcinoid syndrome with gastric carcinoid tumours is similar to that for the small gastrointestinal carcinoids. Like small intestinal carcinoids the gastric tumours have also metastased to the liver by the time the syndrome presents, though epigastric pain, anorexia, weight loss, and gastrointestinal bleeding may present as symptoms of the primary tumour itself. Gastric carcinoids are frequently polypoid but are not apparently located in any specific area of the stomach. Sometimes they are multiple and in the incredible case reported by Black and Haffner (1968), hundreds of small nodules of tumour were present in the gastric wall and there appeared to be a generalized hypertrophy of the enterochromaffin cell system in the stomach, raising the possibility that the activity of the enterochromaffin cell system might be under the control of trophic influences analogous to other endocrine glands. Bony metastases from the gastric tumour are not uncommon and these may be osteosclerotic.

The microscopic appearance of gastric carcinoids is similar to that of other carcinoid tumours but the histochemical reactions are different. The gastric carcinoid is normally negative to argentaffin staining reactions but shows argyrophilia. This different histochemical picture is accompanied by certain frequent clinical and biochemical features suggesting special functional activity. Briefly, geographical flushing is common, as is headache, and the tumours sometimes produce histamine. 5-hydroxytryptophan and 5-hydroxytryptamine as well as 5HIAA may be found in the urine. These aspects are discussed later.

Bronchial Carcinoids

Kramer (1930) first used the term bronchial adenoma to differentiate this type of tumour from the more usual rapidly malignant bronchogenic carcinomas. Weiss and Ingram (1961) have examined carefully this group of tumours and confirm the work of Hamperl (1937) that two major independent types of bronchial neoplasm are included under the heading bronchial adenoma. The difference between these two groups has also been emphasized by Feyrter (1959a, b) and Williams and Azzopardi (1960). The smaller of these two groups is comprised of neoplasms of the salivary gland type, so called adenoid cystic carcinomas (cylindromas) and mucoepidermoid tumours. The larger of the two groups is comprised of bronchial carcinoid tumours and it is these tumours with which the carcinoid syndrome may be associated.

Weiss and Ingram (1961) give the impression that bronchial carcinoids have a low degree of malignancy but Goodner, Berg and Watson (1961) in their series found that in 44% of their entire series of 27 metastases were present. When these tumours produce the carcinoid syndrome it is true to say that distant metastases are usually present (Dockerty *et al.,* 1958; Kincaid Smith and Brossy, 1956; Warner and Southren, 1958; Schneckloth McIsaac and Page, 1959; Weiss and Ingram, 1961). However this is not invariably the case (Von Bernheimer *et al.,* 1964).

Bronchial carcinoids usually arise from the mucosa of major segmental bronchi, lobar or main bronchi. Bronchial carcinoid tumours appear histologically not unlike gastrointestinal carcinoids. However, the morphological pattern may be trabecular, acinar or alveolar and palisading of peripheral cells may be seen. Mucin secretion may occur. One gets the impression that there may be a good deal of pleomorphism in these tumours and that sometimes it can be difficult on histological appearance to definitely diagnose the bronchial carcinoid tumour (Plate 13).

The histochemical reaction of these tumours is variable and this has led to much discussion which it would not be profitable to go into here. Positive argentaffin staining reactions are not as frequent as in gastrointestinal carcinoids. Holley (1946) found only one case out of 30 with argentaffin granules, Feyrter (1959a) 7 out of 19, and Williams and Azzopardi (1960) 4 out of 9. Frequently, however, they give a positive argyrophil reaction (Williams and Azzopardi, 1960). Positive azo-dye coupling seems to be less common than argentaffinity or argyrophilia.

Recent studies by Bensch and his colleagues (1965a, b) and (1968) on the cell of origin of the bronchial carcinoid and the relation between this tumour and the oat cell carcinoma of the bronchus are fascinating and worthy of more detailed examination.

Froehlich (1949) and Feyrter (1953) both observed the presence of cells resembling Kultschitzky cells in the mucosa of bronchi. Bensch *et al.* (1965a) found such a cell wedged between the basal parts of the columna epithelial cells lining the acini and ducts of normal bronchial glands. The cell on electron microscopy contained 'Neurosecreting' granules, little endoplasmic reticulum, relatively clear cytoplasm and pseudopodia which spread into the intercellular spaces among the glandular cells. They found cells of very similar appearance to compose three bronchial carcinoid tumours and they state that undoubtedly these tumours arise from the Kultschitzky-type cell normally but scantily present in bronchial mucosa which is similar in its fine structure with the intestinal argentaffin cell.

Recent observations show that oat cell carcinomas of the bronchus may also on occasion cause the carcinoid syndrome, (Rørvik, 1955; Parish *et al.,* 1964; Gowenlock *et al.,* 1964; Harrison *et al.,* 1957; Azzopardi and Bellan, 1965; Kinloch *et al.,* 1965; Williams and Azzopardi, 1960). In addition, of course, there are now many reports of bronchial oat cell carcinomas producing other hormones such as ACTH, MSH, ADH, parathormone and gonadotrophins (see Liddle, *et al.,* 1969). On occasions too, certain of these endocrine abnormalities may occur in association with the carcinoid syndrome (see Chapter 7). Because of its endocrine potential, Bensch *et al.* (1968) examined electron-microscopically the oat-celled tumour. They found in the cells of these tumours neuro-secreting granules similar to those found in bronchial 'Kultschitzky' cells and in the cells of bronchial carcinoids and in addition found the oat cells to possess pseudopod-like cytoplasmic processes. On the basis of their findings these authors consider that bronchial carcinoids and oat-celled carcinomas of the bronchus both derive from Kultschitzky-type cells normally found in bronchial mucosa. They look upon the bronchial carcinoid as a locally spreading but rather benign neoplasm and the oat-celled carcinoma as the anaplastic highly malignant form of the tumour.

REFERENCES

Anthony, P. P. and Drury, R. A. B. (1970). Elastic vascular sclerosis of mesenteric blood vessels in argentaffin carcinoma. *J. Clin. Path.* **23**, 110.

Askanazy, Von M. (1923). Zur Pathogenese der Magenkrebse und über ihren Gelegentlichenursprung aus angeborenen Epitheliolen Keimen in der Magenward. *Deutsch. Med. Wschr.* **49**, 49.

Azzopardi, J. G. and Bellan, A. R. (1965). Carcinoid syndrome and oat cell carcinoma of the bronchus. *Thorax,* **20,** 393.

Black, W. C. and Haffner, H. E. (1968). Diffuse hyperplasia of gastric argyrophil cells and multiple carcinoid tumours. *Cancer,* **21,** 1080.

Bensch, K. G., Gordon, G. B. and Miller, L. R. (1965a). Studies on bronchial counterpart of the Kultschitzky (argentaffin) cell and innervation of bronchial glands. *J. Ultrastructural Research,* **12,** 668.

Bensch, K. G., Gordon, G. B. and Miller, L. R. (1965b). Electron microscopic and biochemical studies on the bronchial carcinoid tumour. *Cancer,* **18,** 592.

Bensch, K. G., Corrin, B., Pariente, R. and Spencer, H. (1968). Oat cell carcinoma of the lung: its origin and relationship to bronchial carcinoid. *Cancer,* **22,** 1163.

Christodoulopoulos, J. B. and Klotz, A. P. (1961). Carcinoid syndrome with primary carcinoid tumour of the stomach. *Gastroenterology,* **40,** 429.

Dockerty, M. B., McGoon, D. C., Fontana, R. S. and Scudamore, H. H. (1958). Metastasising bronchial carcinoid with hyperserotoninaemia and carcinoid syndrome. Report of a case. *M. Clin. North America,* **42,** 975.

Fein, S. B. and Knudtson, K. P. (1956). The malignant carcinoid syndrome; a case report with biochemical studies. *Cancer,* **9,** 148.

Feyrter, F. (1959a). Uber das bronchuscarcinoid. *Virchows Arch. path. Anat.* **332,** 25.

Feyrter, F. (1959b). Uber das Cylindrom (mucipare Adenom) des Bronchialbaumes. *Virchows, Arch. path. Anat.* **332,** 44.

Foreman, R. C. (1952). Carcinoid Tumours: report of 38 cases. *Ann. Surg.* **136,** 838.

Froehlich, F. (1949). Die 'Helle Zelle' der Bronchialschleimhaut und ihre Beziehungen zum Problem der chemoreceptoren. *Frankf. Z. Path.* **60,** 517.

Goodner, J. T., Berg, J. W. and Watson, W. L. (1961). The non-benign nature of bronchial carcinoids and cylindromas. *Cancer,* **14,** 539.

Gowenlock, A. H., Platt, D. S., Campbell, A. C. P. and Wormsley, K. G. (1964). Oat cell carcinoma of the bronchus secreting 5-hydroxytryptophan. *Lancet,* **1,** 304.

Hamperl, H. (1937). Uber gutartige Bronchial tumouren (Cylindrome und Carcinoide). *Virchows Arch. path. Anat.* **300,** 46.

Harrison, M. T., Montgomery, D. A. D., Ramsey, A. S., Robertson, J. H. and Welbourn, R. B. (1957). Cushing's syndrome with carcinoma of the bronchus and with features suggesting a carcinoid tumour. *Lancet,* **1,** 23.

Holley, S. W. (1946). Bronchial Adenomas. *Milit. Surg.* **99,** 528.

Kincaid-Smith, P. and Brossy, J. J. (1956). Case of bronchial adenoma with liver metastasis. *Thorax.* **11,** 36.

Kinloch, J. D., Webb, J. N., Eccleston, D. and Zeitlin, J. (1965). Carcinoid syndrome associated with oat cell carcinoma of bronchus. *Brit. med. J.* **1,** 1533.

Kramer, R. (1930). Adenoma of bronchus. *Ann. Otol. Rhin. & Laryng.* **39,** 689.

Liddle, G. W., Nicholson, W. E., Island, D. P., Orth, D. N., Abe, K. and Lowder, S. C. (1969). Clinical and laboratory studies of ectopic hormone syndrome. *Recent prog. horm. Research,* **25,** 283.

Lillie, R. D. and Glenner, G. G. (1960). Histochemical reactions in carcinoid tumours of the gastrointestinal tract. *Am. J. Path.* **36,** 623.

Lubasch, O. (1888). Uber den primären Krebs des ileum nebst Bemerkungen uber das gleichzeitige Vorkommen des Krebses und der Tuberkulose. *Virchows Arch. path. Anat.* **111,** 281.

MacDonald, R. A. (1956). Study of 356 carcinoids of the gastrointestinal tract: Report of four new cases of the carcinoid syndrome. *Am. J. Med.* **21**, 867.

Moertel, C. G., Dockerty, M. B. and Baggenstoss, A. H. (1961). Multiple primary malignant neoplasms. I, II and III. *Cancer,* **14**, 221, 231 and 238.

Moertel, C. G., Sauer, W. G., Dockerty, M. B. and Baggenstoss, A. H. (1961). Life history of the carcinoid tumour in the small intestine. *Cancer,* **14**, 901.

Parish, D. J.,Crawford, N. and Spencer, A. T. (1964). The secretion of 5-hydroxytryptamine by a poorly differentiated bronchial carcinoma. *Thorax,* **19**, 62.

Pearse, A. G. E. (1960). *Histochemistry, Theoretical and Applied.* (2nd ed.). Churchill, London.

Pearson, C. M. and Fitzgerald, P. J. (1949). Carcinoid Tumours: re-empahses of their malignant nature: review of 140 cases. *Cancer,* **2**, 1005.

Pochaczeosky, R. and Sherman, R. S. (1959). The roentgen appearance of gastric argentaffinoma. *Radiology,* **72**, 330.

Pollock, A. V. (1959). Relief of flushing after resection of a secreting argentaffinoma. *Brit. J. Surg.* **46**, 543.

Rørvik, K. (1955). Malignant intestinal carcinoid and vasomotor disturbances. *J. Oslo City Hosp.* **5**, 133.

Sauer, W. G., Dearing, W. H., Flock, E. V., Waugh, J. M., Dockerty, M. B. and Roth, G. M. (1958). Functioning carcinoid tumours. *Gastroenterology,* **34**, 216.

Sander, R. J. and Axtell, H. K. (1964). Carcinoids of the gastrointestinal tract. *Surg. Gynec. Obstet.* **199**, 369.

Sandler, M. (1968). 5-hydroxyindoles and the carcinoid syndrome. *Adv. Pharmacol.* **6B**, 127.

Sandler, M. and Snow, P. J. D. (1958). An atypical carcinoid tumour secreting 5-hydroxytryptophan. *Lancet.* **1**, 137.

Schneckloth, R. E., McIsaac, W. M. and Page, I. H. (1959). Serotonin metabolism in carcinoid syndrome with metastatic bronchial adenoma. *JAMA.* **170**, 1143.

Von Bernheimer, H., Ehnriger, H., Heistracher, P., Kraupp, P., Lachnit, V., Obiditsch-Mayer, I. and Wenzl, M. (1960). Biologisch aktives, nicht metastasiergendes Bronchuscarcinoid mit Linksherzsyndrom. *Wien. klin. Wchnschr.* **72**, 867.

Warner, R. R. P. and Southren, A. L. (1958). Carcinoid syndrome produced by metastasising bronchial adenoma. *Am. J. Med.* **24**, 903.

Warren, K. W. and Coyle, E. B. Carcinoid tumours of gastrointestinal tract. *Am. J. Surg.* **82**, 372.

Weiss, L. and Ingram, M. (1961). Adenomatoid bronchial tumours. Two major independent types. *Cancer,* **14**, 161.

Williams, E. D. and Azzopardi, J. G. (1960). Tumours of the lung and the carcinoid syndrome. *Thorax,* **15**, 30.

Williams, E. D. and Sandler, M. (1963). The classification of carcinoid tumours. *Lancet.* **1**, 238.

Wilson, H., Storer, E. H. and Starr, F. J. (1963). Carcinoid tumours; a study of 78 cases. *Am. J. Surg.* **105**, 35.

CHAPTER 4

Biochemistry

5-hydroxytryptamine

Erspamer and his colleagues (see Erspamer, 1954) over a period of nineteen years sought to identify a substance with many potent pharmacological properties, which they called 'Enteramine', and which they found in tumours containing enterochromaffin cells in many species. In the final study of characterization of this material (Erspamer and Asero, 1953), 30 kg of posterior salivary gland tissue removed from 30,000. octopuses (*Octopus vulgaris*) and the skin from 1020 Sicilian amphibians (*Discoglossous pictus*) were used. From both these sources enteramine was purified as its picrate salt, chemically characterized as 5-hydroxytryptamine and found to be identical with authentic synthesized 5-hydroxytryptamine (Asero *et al.*, 1952).

During the later stages of this work, Rapport *et al.* (1948) had independently been studying the nature of the substance responsible for the vasoconstricting property of serum (O'Connor, 1912). Rapport and his colleagues named this substance 'Serotonin' and from beef serum a substance was isolated which by various chemical criteria was thought to be the creatinine sulphate salt of 5-hydroxytryptamine (Rapport, 1949). When Hamlin and Fisher (1951) synthesized 5-hydroxytryptamine it was evident that Rapport had been correct in the structure he had assigned to 'Serotonin'. It was not until 1952, however, that it became apparent that Enteramine and Serotonin were identical.

When the structure of 5-hydroxytryptamine became known work began on its mode of biosynthesis and metabolism. Three routes for its biosynthesis were considered:

1. The 5-hydroxylation of tryptamine formed by the decarboxylation of tryptophan.
2. The 5-hydroxylation of tryptophan with the formation of 5-hydroxytryptophan which is then decarboxylated to form 5-hydroxytryptamine.
3. The cyclization of 2:5-dihydroxyphenylalanine to form 5-hydroxyindole with subsequent insertion of the β-ethylamine side chain.

Using 5-hydroxytryptophan synthesized by Ek and Witkop (1953), Udenfriend *et. al.* (1953) showed that homogenates of guinea pig kidney enzymatically decarbocylated 5-hydroxytryptophan to form 5-hydroxytryptamine. The same group of workers partially purified the enzyme and demonstrated its requirement for pyridoxal phosphate (Clark *et al.,* 1954). At first the decarboxylation was thought to be specific for 5HTP, but Lovenberg *et al.* (1962) have shown that the enzyme prepared from guinea pig kidney, brain and intestine will decarboxylate the L-isomers of dihydroxyphenylalanine, 5-hydroxy-tryptophan, tyrosine, phenylalanine, tryptophan and to a small degree histidine. Hagen (1960) has questioned whether all similar de-carboxylases have such a wide specificity, demonstrating that decarboxylases prepared from carcinoid tumours and phaeochromo-cytomas will decarboxylate 5-hydroxytryptophan and DOPA but not other aromatic amino acids.

Blaschko (1952) demonstrated that 5-hydroxytryptamine was oxidatively deaminated by guinea pig tissues and Titus and Udenfriend (1954) observed that the end metabolic product of this oxidative deamination was 5-hydroxyindole acetic acid. Weissbach *et al.* (1957) found the direct product of oxidative deamination to be 5-hydroxyin-dole acetaldehyde, this being converted to 5-hydroxyindole acetic acid by alcohol dehydrogenase.

The position was reached therefore where it seemed possible that the route of synthesis of 5-hydroxytryptamine was via 5-hydroxytryptophan and of metabolism to 5-hydroxyindole acetic acid. 5-hydroxytryptophan is not an amino acid abundant in nature and has to be synthesized by an animal requiring it. Because of this, Udenfriend *et al.* (1956) carried out a series of important experiments. They utilized the toad, Bufo Marinus, the venom glands of which contain large amounts of 5-hydroxy-N-methyl-tryptamine, N-N-dimethyl-5-hydroxytryptamine (Bufotenine), β-[5-hydroxy-indolyl-(3)]-ethyl) trimethylammonium hydroxide (Bufo-tenidine) as well as 5-hydroxytryptamine. Radioactive tryptophan was administered to the toad and the radioactive label was recovered in these 5-hydroxyindoles, and in particular 5-hydroxytryptophan became labelled. In addition, the administration of radioactive tryptophan to rabbits led to labelling of the 5-hydroxytryptamine bound to platelets. Udenfriend *et al.* (1956) also administered tryptophan-2-C^{14} to a patient with carcinoid syndrome and showed that the urinary 5-hydroxyindole acetic acid became radioactive. That the carcinoid tumour was dependent upon a supply of tryptophan for the synthesis of 5-hydroxytryptamine was shown in the investigations of Smith *et al.* (1957) where the urinary level of 5HIAA rose and fell *pari passu* with the amount of tryptophan in the diet. Scattered observations supported the evidence that 5-hydroxytryptophan was the intermediate in the conversion of tryptophan to 5-hydroxytryptamine. Dalgleish (1956) and Sandler and Snow (1958) identified 5-hydroxytryptophan in the urine of certain patients with the carcinoid syndrome. Donaldson *et al.* (1959) administered radioactive tryptophan to a patient with the carcinoid syndrome where urine contained 5-hydroxytryptophan and found that this substance became radioactive.

Tryptamine was ruled out as a physiological precursor of 5-hydroxytryptamine by the investigations of Udenfriend *et al.* (1959). Likewise, the administration of radioactive phenylalanine and tyrosine to the toad did not lead to labelling of the 5-hydroxyindoles in the venom sacs, excluding 2.5-dihydroxyphenylalanine as a precursor.

The evidence therefore pointed to the sequence shown in Figure 1 as being the physiological route of 5-hydroxytryptamine biosynthesis in animal tissues.

However, the enzymatic conversion of tryptophan to 5-hydroxytryptophan proved difficult to demonstrate. Mitoma *et al.* (1956) demonstrated this reaction in a bacterium, Chromobacterium Violaceum, an organism which makes a pigment Violacein, this pigment containing a 5-hydroxyindole structure (Beer *et al.*, 1954). This activity could not be demonstrated, however, when the bacteria were broken. Schindler (1958) incubated neoplastic mast cells containing 5-hydroxytryptamine, with radioactive tryptophan and was able to demonstrate the conversion of tryptophan to 5-hydroxytryptamine. 5-hydroxytryptophan was not identified as an intermediate however. Cooper and Melcer (1961) reported the synthesis of 5-hydroxytryptamine from tryptophan in cell free preparations of rat intestinal mucosa.

In 1961, Freedland *et al.* were able to demonstrate that preparations of rat liver 5-hydroxylated tryptophan but Renson *et al.* (1962) showed that this activity was due to the phenylalanine hydroxylase activity of the liver and was not a physiological mechanism for the biosynthesis of 5-hydroxytryptamine.

Because in the carcinoid syndrome there is an increased synthesis of 5-hydroxytryptamine, I chose to examine carcinoid tumours and their metastases to study *in vitro* their ability to hydroxylate tryptophan with the formation of 5-hydroxytryptophan and to complete the pathway to form 5-hydroxytryptamine (Grahame-Smith, 1964, 1967a, b). It was possible to demonstrate in slices of carcinoid tumours and their metastases removed both at autopsy and at operation the enzymatic conversion of L-tryptophan to L-5-hydroxytryptophan and the conversion of the latter to 5-hydroxytryptamine (see Table 7). The enzyme converting L-tryptophan to L-5-hydroxytryptophan (tryptophan 5-hydroxylase) was partially purified from preparations of carcinoid tumour and the enzyme was shown to require a reduced pteridine cofactor for full activity. The enzyme isolated from the carcinoid

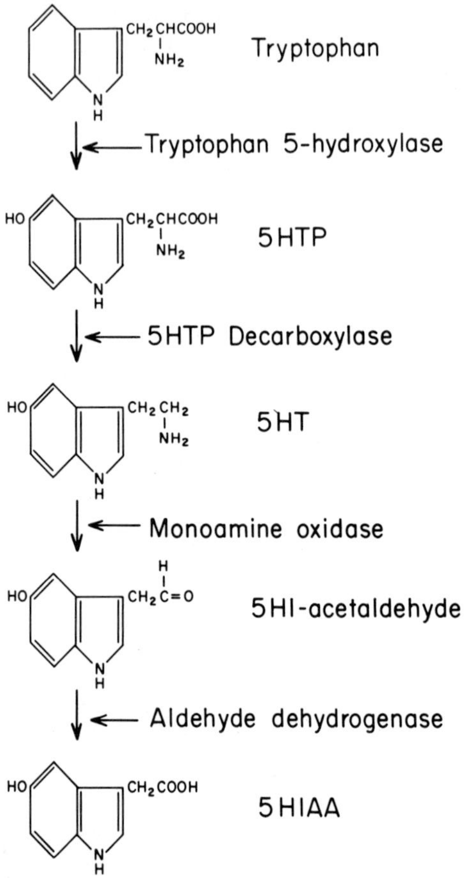

CH₂CHCOOH
Tryptophan

Tryptophan 5-hydroxylase

5HTP

5HTP Decarboxylase

5HT

Monoamine oxidase

5HI-acetaldehyde

Aldehyde dehydrogenase

5HIAA

Fig. 1. The synthesis and metabolism of 5-hydroxytryptamine. 5HTP = 5-hydroxytryptophan; 5HT = 5-hydroxytryptamine; 5HI acetaldehyde = 5-hydroxyindole acetaldehyde; 5HIAA = 5-hydroxyindole acetic acid. The 5-hydroxyindoles shown above are the most important in understanding the involvement of serotonin in the carcinoid syndrome.

tumour proved to be different from the phenylalanine hydroxylase in liver but is probably similar in some respects to that subsequently demonstrated in brain (Grahame-Smith, 1967), pineal gland (Lovenberg *et al.*, 1967) and normal intestine (Grahame-Smith, 1967a). A comparison of the activity of the carcinoid tumour to synthesize 5-hydroxytryptamine, with the activity of brain and intestinal preparations, suggested that the increased biosynthesis of 5-hydroxyindoles in the carcinoid syndrome is due to a greatly increased number of functional cells and not due to an increased function of individual cells (Grahame-Smith, 1967a). Tryptophan hydroxylation has been dealt with in some detail because this is the rate-limiting enzymatic reaction in the synthesis of 5-hydroxytryptamine. The subsequent decarboxylation of 5-hydroxytryptophan is not rate-limiting and indeed the decarboxylase is widespread and active in many tissues including most (Langemann, 1958) but not all (Campbell *et al.,* 1963) carcinoid tumours.

THE EFFECT OF DMPH$_4$ UPON THE ACTIVITY OF TRYPTOPHAN

5-HYDROXYLASE PARTIALLY PURIFIED FROM TUMOUR

Addition	Carrier 5HTP added (μ mole)	5HT recovered (μ mole)	Specific activity of recovered 5HT (c/m/μ mole)	μμmole 5HTP produced/ hr/ml of preparation
None	4	0.089	2×10^3	49
DMPH$_4$(2 mM)	4	0.065	1.88×10^4	525

Table 7. The synthesis of 5HT by a carcinoid tumour. Hepatic metastases from an ileal argentaffinoma were homogenized. The non-particulate matter was separated by centrifugation and a protein fraction from this precipitated with ammonium sulphate. This protein precipitate was taken and redissolved and dialysed to remove the ammonium sulphate. Aliquots of the protein fraction were then incubated with radioactive tryptophan-C14, in the presence or absence of a reduced pteridine co-factor (5,6,7,8-tetrahydro-6,7-dimethylpteridine). At the end of the incubation non-radioactive 5-hydroxytryptophan was added as a carrier and the 5-hydroxytryptophan was separated by paper chromatography and high voltage paper electrofluorescis. The 5-hydroxytryptophan was then taken and decarboxylated with an aromatic amino acid decarboxylase preparation and the 5-hydroxytryptamine formed was isolated by paper chromatography and its specific activity was measured and the recovery calculated. As can be seen from this table the reduced pteridine co-factor was necessary for full activity of the enzyme.

As already mentioned, the chief route of metabolism of 5-hydroxytryptamine is by oxidative deamination to 5-hydroxyindole acetic acid. The studies of Page *et al.* (1956) established excessive urinary excretion of 5-hydroxyindole acetic acid as the biochemical hallmark of the carcinoid syndrome. Many other routes of metabolism are in fact available to 5-hydroxytryptamine (see Garattini and Valzelli, 1966), but none of these appears to be of quantitative importance except perhaps the conversion to 5-hydroxytryptophol (Davis *et al.,* 1966, 1967;

Feldstein, 1967). When 5-hydroxytryptamine undergoes oxidative deamination the first product is 5-hydroxyindole acetaldehyde. When ethanol is ingested there appears to be increased metabolism of 5-hydroxyindole acetaldehyde to 5-hydroxytryptophol, away from 5-hydroxyindole acetic acid. The main pathways of biosynthesis and metabolism of 5-hydroxytryptamine are shown in Fig. 1.

Having discussed the main points concerning the biochemistry of 5-hydroxytryptamine it is necessary to consider these in the context of the carcinoid syndrome and its causative tumour.

Normally only about 1% of the 0.5-1.0 G of dietary tryptophan intake is converted to 5-hydroxytryptamine, the rest being metabolized by other routes, mainly via the kyneurinine pathway, by decarboxylation to tryptamine, and also by incorporation into protein. In the carcinoid syndrome the tumour seems able to take up tryptophan avidly since 5-hydroxyindole acetic acid excretion may rise from the normal of less than 10 mg/day to over 500 mg/day. Thus the amount of tryptophan utilized for 5-hydroxyindole synthesis may increase from 1% to over 50%. This may lead to a low concentration of tryptophan in the plasma. In six recorded cases plasma tryptophan levels were low in five (Sjoerdsma *et al.*, 1956; Sjoerdsma *et al.*, 1957). In the cases studied at St Mary's, four cases out of five have had definitely low plasma tryptophan levels. One might expect urinary tryptophan levels to be low. However, on the evidence of urinary paper chromatography there is little evidence for this since one can usually find in patients with the syndrome what appears to be a fairly normal amount of urinary tryptophan. Tryptophan deficiency may manifest itself by nicotinamide deficiency. Nicotinamide is synthesized from tryptophan and patients with the syndrome may excrete diminished amounts of N-methylnicotinamide (Sjoerdsma *et al.*, 1957), and also show signs of pellagra.

Tryptophan on being taken into the tumour is 5-hydroxylated to form 5-hydroxytryptophan by tryptophan 5-hydroxylase. This reaction, as already mentioned, requires a reduced pteridine cofactor. It is of interest that intestinal mucosa and argentaffin tumours were shown many years ago (Jacobson and Simpson, 1946) to contain pteridines, particularly Xanthopterin. These substances are presumably synthesized from folic acid. As far as I am aware, there is no reported increased incidence of folate deficient megaloblastic anaemia in the carcinoid syndrome, which might be expected if there were overall folic acid deficiency due to excessive usage of it by the tumour. Tryptophan hydroxylation in several tissues (see Koe and Weissman, 1966) can be inhibited by p-chlorophenylalanine and this compound is effective in inhibiting tryptophan hydroxylation in the carcinoid tumour (Englemann *et al.*, 1967). The clinical usage and effects of this drug are further discussed on page 77.

Little work has been done on the subcellular localization of tryptophan hydroxylase in the carcinoid tumour. In one tumour which has been studied the tryptophan hydroxylase activity sedimented with particulate matter in a cell free homogenate (Grahame-Smith, 1968). Such matters are not of purely academic interest since the spatial organization within the cell of the hydroxylation and the 5-hydroxytryptophan produced, the decarboxylation and the 5-hydroxytryptophan produced, the decarboxylation and the 5-hydroxytryptamine produced and the storage mechanism for 5-hydroxytryptamine must be of importance for the overall functional integrity of the system, yet how little we know of the intracellular spatial organization of such systems.

In the typical mid-gut carcinoid the 5-hydroxytryptophan produced is decarboxylated to 5-hydroxytryptamine. These tumours contain the decarboxylase. However, it appears that in some tumours arising from fore-gut derivatives, i.e. bronchus, stomach and pancreas, 5-hydroxytryptophan is released from the tumour, some of which is probably decarboxylated at other sites in the body leading to the appearance of 5-hydroxytryptophan, 5-hydroxytryptamine and 5-hydroxyindole acetic acid in the urine (Oates and Sjoerdsma, 1962). This release of the precursor of 5-hydroxytryptamine, 5-hydroxytryptophan which is normally not even detectable in mid-gut tumours (Gowenlock and Platt, 1960) because of the great activity of the decarboxylase, could be due either to faulty organization of the biosynthetic process so that 5-hydroxytryptophan is released rather than being decarboxylated or to a true lack or inactivity of the decarboxylase. Campbell *et al.* (1963) have investigated one such tumour. It contained low levels of 5-hydroxytryptamine but appreciable amounts of 5HTP. This tumour contained no detectable decarboxylase, so it looks as if decarboxylase lack is responsible for the biochemical variant. Is this lack characteristic of the cell from which these tumours arise? It seems unlikely that this is simply due to aberrant biochemical differentiation undergone during carcinogenesis since if this were so why is it that mid-gut carcinoids rarely show this abnormality? On the other hand, if this is not so, then it would imply that the cell of origin lacks the decarboxylase and this, in a cell able to hydroxylate tryptophan, would be a very strange state of affairs. The truth of this matter cannot yet be stated. Certainly, however, the unusual pattern of 5-hydroxyindoles in the urine of these atypical cases does seem to be due to 5-hydroxytryptophan release by the tumour since infusions of 5HTP (Oates and Sjoerdsma, 1962) and the administration of α-methyldopa to carcinoid patients, a substance which partially inhibits 5HTP decarboxylase, produce a similar urinary pattern.

In the more typical ileal tumours 5HTP is decarboxylated to 5HT. The 5HT is then stored in the tumour, 5HTP usually being undetectable on paper chromatography of extracts. The actual amounts found in the tumour vary greatly. This must depend upon rates of synthesis, storage and release and intra-tumour metabolism by monoamine oxidase found in the tumour (Langemann, 1958) and cellularity. However, Gowenlock and Platt (1960) reviewing the literature, find values which vary very much. As a guide, though ileal primary tumours may contain as much as 1420 μg/G (wet weight) 5HT or as little as 15 μg/G, of 38 tumours reviewed and of 58 tissue analyses done 47 showed levels less than 1000 μg/G and 22 under 500 μg/G. Zeitlhofer and Formanek (1959) found the incredibly high level of 7 mg/G in a post mortem mediastinal secondary tumour. Metastatic tumours in liver, lymph nodes and elsewhere also contain large quantities of 5HT and retain the capacity to synthesize it. There is no fixed relationship between the concentration of 5HT in the tumour and the degree of increase in urinary 5HIAA. In fact there are notable anomalies, for instance that of Gowenlock and Platt (1960) where the primary contained 1420 μg 5HT/G and the urinary 5HIAA was apparently normal.

Bronchial carcinoids tend to contain lower concentrations of 5HT than ileal tumours, from 250 μg/G (Bernheimer et al., 1960), which is high for tumours in this site, to more usual levels of up to about 50-80 μg/G. Other bronchial tumours such as oat-celled carcinomas associated with syndrome also contain 5HT, the case of Williams and Azzopardi (1960) containing 20 μg/G 5HT with urinary 5HIAA of 64 mg/24 h.

The ovarian carcinoids found in ovarian teratomas may contain large amounts of 5HT, 432 μg/G (Pernow and Waldenström, 1957), 2120 μg/G (Sauer et al., 1958).

Gastric carcinoids and their metastases tend to contain rather low quantities of 5HT, e.g. 0.33 μg/G (Snow et al. Lancet, 1958) and may also contain 5HTP.

Not a great deal of investigation has been done on the mechanism by which 5HT is stored in these tumours and this in fact is part of a larger problem of the mechanism of storage of pharmacologically active substances, particularly the monoamines, adrenaline and noradrenaline, histamine and 5HT. In sites in which one or other of these amines are found, nerve endings (catecholamines and 5HT), adrenal medulla (catecholamines), mast cells (histamine and 5HT), platelets (5HT), the monoamines appear to be stored partly in association with granules. This is so in the normal argentaffin cell and electron microscopic studies make it plain that similar storage granules are present in the cells of carcinoid tumours. Prusoff (1960) has shown that cytoplasmic granules can be isolated from normal gastrointestinal mucosal homogenates by density gradient centrifugation and that 5HT is associated with them. Such granules also contain ATP in high concentration on a molar ration of 2.6 : 1. This association also exists in platelets for 5HT and ATP and in normal adrenal medullary tissue and phaeochromocytoma tissue for adrenaline, noradrenaline and ATP (Blaschko *et al.,* 1968). These latter workers have also found a specific protein, chromogranin, in adrenal medullary granules and it is suggested that this protein and ATP are in some way necessary for the storage of the catecholamines. It is likely that a similar mechanism is operative for 5HT but insufficient work has been done to say whether this is so or not.

Recently, Dr David Smith (Department of Pharmacology, University of Oxford) and I have studied hepatic metastases removed at operation from a patient with a primary ileal carcinoid tumour. We found that 5HT was bound to granular fraction but that in fact these granules contained little ATP (Fig. 2). The nature of the binding of 5HT to argentaffin granules is still a subject for further investigation.

Although 5HT is synthesized and stored by carcinoid tumours it is equally apparent that it is released. The work of Robertson *et al.* (1961), however, showed that in the majority of patients during paroxysmal flushing there was no paroxysmal release of 5HT (though, as will be discussed later, Oates *et al.* (1964) have shown paroxysmal release of kallikrein). In the series studied by Robertson *et al.* (1961) there was an important exception. This patient, a female aged 58 with an ileal carcinoid with metastases and the syndrome, was shown to have paroxysmal release of 5HT, accompanied by hyperventilation and a cyanotic flush in response to noradrenaline, so that in certain patients such release may occur. Even without paroxysmal release, however, the evidence that intact 5HT enters the circulation is incontrovertible, since whole blood levels of 5HT are frequently raised.

Whole blood 5HT lies in the range of 0.1-0.3 μg/ml (see Gowenlock and Platt, 1960). Because platelets contain large quantities of 5HT and are avid for this substance which they take up both *in vivo* and *in vitro,* the free plasma levels are considerably lower, 0.02-0.04 μg/ml (see Gowenlock and Platt, 1960), but these are difficult to measure because of the difficulty of preventing platelet disruption in the process of preparing platelet free plasma. Gowenlock *et al.,* reviewing whole blood 5HT levels, found this to be elevated in 25 out of 27 cases. Robertson *et al.* (1961), however, found the free plasma 5HT not to be much raised, varying from 0.06 to 0.075 μg/ml of platelet free plasma in the resting state (non-flushing). The situation in most patients seems to be like this. 5HT is probably only slowly released and probably not paroxysmally in the majority of patients. The mechanism of this release is unknown, though some headway has been made in understanding the release mechanism in the case of kallikrein. What happens to 5HT which is released? Vane (1969) believes that binding to platelets is relatively unimportant. It appears that the lung is functionally important in inactivating by uptake several humoral substances. Apparently the lung

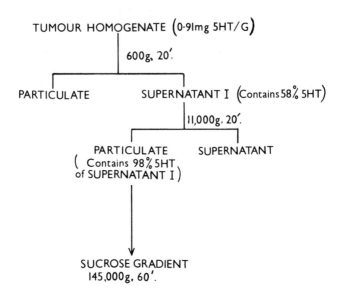

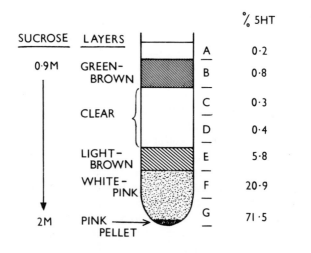

Fig. 2. The distribution of serotonin in subcellular fractions prepared from hepatic metastases of an ileal argentaffinoma. Hepatic metastases were homogenized and after separation of the nuclei, an 11,000 G particulate fraction was layered on a discontinuous density gradient of sucrose. On such a gradient particulate matter according to its density will sink through the gradient to an equilibrium point. As shown above most of the serotonin was found in fraction G. The ATP content of this fraction was < 48 μg/mg 5HT which gives a molar ratio of 5HT : ATP of > 33.

does not metabolize much of the 5HT by oxidative deamination but perhaps hands on the 5HT to platelets.

Davis (1968) has shown that in carcinoid patients the ability of the lung to take up 5HT varies and this would obviously affect the amount of 5HT entering the systemic circulation. Such factors may be of importance in explaining the variability of symptoms. If 5HT does get into the circulation, and even if bound to platelets which sooner or later must give it up to tissue binding sites, then oxidative metabolism in many tissues occurs with the production of 5HIAA which is excreted. It is important to note, however, that carcinoid tumours themselves contain quite high activities of monoamine oxidase and that 5HIAA can be produced within the tumour and secreted into the blood so that the urinary 5HIAA may reflect not only circulating 5HT oxidatively deaminated outside the tumour, but also 5HIAA released from the tumour. This might also be an explanation why some tumours contain low concentrations of 5HT; perhaps the storage mechanism which protects 5HT from tumour MAO is defective in these tumours and the 5HT is metabolized. If indeed 5HT is avidly bound to platelets and free plasma 5HT is normal or only just raised, then it is difficult to see just how 5HT can cause symptoms. The fact is that we are unaware of how platelets give up their 5HT to tissues and whether or not this is a physiological occurrence. The mechanisms the body has for protecting itself against circulating free 5HT are quite remarkable. Absorption into platelets, inactivation by lung and liver and destruction by tissue monoamine oxidase obviously protects the body largely from its action. Certainly these mechanisms suggest that 5HT is a locally acting hormone except in pathological states such as the carcinoid syndrome.

Oxidative deamination is the main route of metabolic breakdown, but more recently the conversion of 5HT to 5-hydroxytryptophol has been reported (Davis *et al.*, 1966; 1967), and confirmed (Feldstein, 1967). When 5HT undergoes oxidative deamination by monoamine oxidase the first product is 5-hydroxyindole acetaldehyde. When ethanol is ingested in the carcinoid syndrome, 5HIAA excretion falls and 5-hydroxytryptophol excretion rises. Apparently the ethanol causes a diversion of 5-hydroxyindole acetaldehyde to the alcohol. It is not yet known whether the diversion has any part to play in the flush provoking properties of ethanol.

Because examination of the urine is so important in the diagnosis of the carcinoid syndrome, it is worth while considering in some detail the 5-hydroxyindoles which appear in increased quantities. There is considerable variation in the increase in urinary 5HIAA not only from patient to patient but in individual patients from time to time. Gowenlock and Platt (1960) found that more than half the cases of the syndrome have a 5HIAA excretion of greater than 150 mg/24 h

(Normal = 0-10 mg/24 h). Only six patients with the syndrome had levels of less than 20 mg/24 h. There are a very few cases of the syndrome reported with apparently normal 5HIAA excretion (see Sandler, 1968), but these are rare and at present unexplained. Other metabolites of 5HT may appear in the urine; N-acetyl 5HT (McIssac and Page, 1959), 5HT glucuronide 5-hydroxyindole aceturic acid and also the conjugates of 5HIAA, the O-sulphate and ethyl ester. Other unidentified 5-hydroxy-indoles also frequently occur in carcinoid tissue (see Gowenlock and Platt, 1960).

Urinary 5HT

Urinary 5HT excretion is frequently raised though the quantitative measurement of urinary 5HT is not easy. It is only in fore-gut and atypical tumours that it is easily detectable on routine paper chromatography of the urine, and then it is usually in association with 5-hydroxytryptophan. More careful analysis revealed an elevated level in 12 out of 15 cases of carcinoid tumours, two cases had a normal level and in one none was detected (see Gowenlock and Platt, 1960). There is no certain correlation with the urinary increase in 5HIAA excretion. Usually 5HT excretion is less than 1% of the urinary 5HIAA level.

Bradykinin

The work of Robertson *et al.* (1961), Levine and Sjoerdsma (1963) and Oates *et al.* (1964) demonstrated conclusively that 5HT was not the sole cause of carcinoid flushing. Oates and his colleagues noting that catecholamines, which promote carcinoid flushing, also promote the release of kallikrein and formation of bradykinin in the salivary gland (Hilton and Lewis, 1956), studied the role which this vasodilating polypeptide might have in the carcinoid syndrome (see page 47).

Bradykinin is a nonapeptide of the basic structure:

Arg. Pro. Pro. Gly. Phe. Ser. Pro. Phe. Arg.

In addition, lysyl-bradykinin and methionyl-lysyl-bradykinin are natural vasoactive kinins.

These polypeptides are formed enzymically by the action of proteolytic enzyme, kallikrein, upon a substrate kininogen, an α_2-globulin, from which the kinin is cleaved (see Fig. 3). There are two forms of kallikrein (Lewis, 1968). One is a normal plasma constituent present in an inactive form and which has to be 'activated' before enzymatic activity occurs. The other is a glandular kallikrein secreted by exocrine glands such as the salivary glands. In the salivary glands the kallikrein forms kinin from extracellular kininogen and the kinin causes local glandular vasodilatation aiding secretion. On the basis of its physiochemical characteristics the carcinoid kallikrein is more similar to glandular than to plasma kallikrein. Melmon *et al.* (1965), incubated carcinoid kallikrein with purified human kininogen and demonstrated that the main peptide formed was lysyl-bradykinin. In the circulation this would be converted by plasma amino peptidase to bradykinin. Both

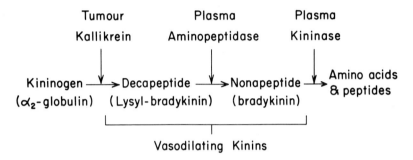

Fig. 3. Scheme of the synthesis and metabolism of bradykinin.

these peptides are vasodilatory and both are converted to smaller inactive peptides by plasma peptidases. But inactivation enzymically is not the only method of inactivation of kinins. Vane (1968) has discussed the role of the lungs and liver in the inactivation of bradykinin and the half life of bradykinin in activating blood appears to be about 17 s. This accords with the short episode of flushing (about 1 min) which occurs when 60 μg bradykinin are given intravenously to man and also with the usually short lived nature of the carcinoid flush. However, carcinoid flushes can last for hours or days, and presumably the length of flush will depend upon the time relationships of the secretion of kallikrein by the tumour.

In those patients who during a flush show a rise in plasma bradykinin levels the sequence of events is presumably:

1. Paroxysmal release of kallikrein from the tumour.
2. Action of kallikrein within the circulating blood to convert kininogen to lysyl-bradykinin.
3. Conversion of lysyl-bradykinin to bradykinin.
4. Action of bradykinin to give vasodilatation.
5. Concurrent destruction of bradykinin by plasma peptidases (kininases) and its tissue inactivation.

There is not much information on how kallikrein is synthesized and stored by carcinoid tumours. Lembeck and his colleagues, however, (see Blaschko, 1968) have found kallikrein in homogenates of the intestinal mucosa in the same intracellular fraction as 5HT. Further studies are awaited on the relationship between 5HT and kallikrein in the argentaffin cell.

Histamine

Some patients, particularly with gastric carcinoid tumours, present with an atypical syndrome. The flush is vivid red and patchy, the latter being very striking. Waldenström *et al.* (1956) sudied one of these patients and showed that as well as increased 5-hydroxyindole production there was an increased amount of histamine in blood and urine. Sandler and Snow (1958) also studied a patient with a gastric primary tumour with atypical 'geographical' flushing and 5HTP in the urine, and found an increased urinary excretion of histamine. Oates and Sjoerdsma (1962) reviewed this situation and found an increased histamine excretion in 4 out of 14 patients studied. In two of these cases the site of the primary tumour was unknown, one was ileal and the other gastric. Urinary histamine excretion is normally 23-90 $\mu g/24$ h and levels up to 4.5 mg/24 h were found in one of their cases.

Although Felberg and Smith (1953) showed that 5HT could release tissue histamine in some species, Oates and Sjoerdsma (1962) could find no evidence for this in man. Waldenström (1956) could find no evidence for a histamine releasing substance in tumour tissue but Campbell *et al.* (1963) were able to show an increased histamine concentration in a gastric carcinoid (105 $\mu g/G$). Increased histamine excretion in these patients may be intermittent (Gowenlock *et al.*, 1964). It seems very likely that the increased circulating histamine and urinary excretion in these patients is due to the ability of the tumour to synthesize it. The known ability of the gastric mucosa to synthesize histamine (Kahlson *et al.*, 1964) and the frequency with which gastric carcinoids secrete histamine fit together and suggests that gastric carcinoids probably derive from the cells which normally synthesize and secrete histamine, in addition to 5HT and kallikrein! The synthesis of histamine is shown in Fig. 4. The enzyme histidine decarboxylase is different from aromatic amino acid decarboxylase, the latter having a very poor activity for decarboxylating histamine (Lovenberg *et al.*, 1962). Gastric mucosa on the other hand contains a histamine decarboxylase and that this enzyme

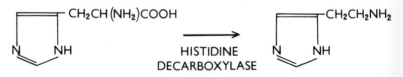

Fig. 4. The scheme of the synthesis of histamine.

is different is further suggested by the fact that while many gastric carcinoids produce histamine they seem unable to effectively decarboxylate 5HTP.

Histamine is metabolized enzymatically to methylhistamine, 1,4-methylimidazole acetic acid and imidazole acetic acid. These substances as well as histamine may appear in the urine of patients with gastric carcinoids (Granérus *et al.*, 1966).

REFERENCES

Asero, B., Colo, V., Erspamer, V. and Vercellone, A. (1952). Synthese des Enteramines (5-Oxytryptamine). *Ann. Chem.* **576**, 69.

Beer, R. J. S., Jennings, B. E. and Robertson, A. (1954). The chemistry of bacteria. Part III. An indolpyrrylmethene from Violacein. *J. Chem. Soc.* 2679.

Bernheimer *et al.* (1960). Biologisch aktives, nicht metastasierendes bronchus-carcinoid mit Linksherzsyndrom. *Wein Klin. Wchnschr.* **72**, 867.

Blaschko, H. (1952). Enzymic oxidation of 5-hydroxytryptamine in mammalian and cephalopod tissue. *Biochem. J.* **52**, 10P.

Blaschko, H. (1968). Reporter's remarks. *Adv. Pharmacol.* **6B**, 205.

Campbell, A. C. P., Gowenlock, A. H., Platt, D. S., Snow, P. J. D. (1963). A 5-hydroxytryptophan secreting carcinoid tumour. *Gut,* **4**, 61.

Clark, C. T., Weissbach, H. and Udenfriend, S. (1954). 5-hydroxytryptophan decarboxylase: preparation and properties. *J. Biol. Chem.* **210**, 139.

Cooper, J. R. and Melcer, I. (1961). The enzymatic conversion of tryptophan to 5-hydroxytryptophan in the biosynthesis of serotonin. *J. Pharmacol. and Exptl. Therap.* **132**, 265.

Davis, V. E., Cashaw, J. L., Huff, J. A. and Brown, H. (1966). Identification of 5-hydroxytryptophol as a serotonin metabolite in man. *Proc. Soc. Exptl. Biol. Med.* **122**, 890.

Davis, V. E., Brown, H., Huff, J. A. and Cashaw, J. L. (1967). The alteration of serotonin metabolism to 5-hydroxytryptophol by ethanol ingestion in man. *J. Lab. Clin. Med.* **69**, 132.

Dalgleish, C. E. (1956). Two-dimensional paper chromatography of urinary indoles and related substances. *Biochem. J.* **64**, 481.

Davis, V. E. (1968). Discussion of the role of 5-hydroxyindoles in the carcinoid syndrome. *Adv. Pharmacol.* **6B**, 143.

Donaldson, R. M., Gray, S. J. and Letson, V. G. (1959). 5-hydroxytryptophan as an intermediate of serotonin biosynthesis in malignant carcinoidoses. *Lancet,* **2**, 1002.

Ek, A. and Witkop, B. (1953). Synthesis and biochemistry of 5- and 7-hydroxytryptophan and derivatives. *J. Am. Chem. Soc.* **75**, 500.

Engleman, K., Lovenberg, W. and Sjoerdsma, A. (1967). Inhibition of serotonin synthesis by para-chlorophenylalanine in patients with the carcinoid syndrome. *New. Eng. J. Med.* **277**, 1103.

Erspamer, V. (1954). The pharmacology of indolealkylamines. *Pharmacol. rev.* **6**, 425.

Erspamer, V. and Asero, B. (1953). Isolation of enteramine from extracts of posterior salivary glands of *Octopus vulgaris* and of *Discoglossus pictus* skin. *J. Biol. Chem.* **200**, 311.

Feldberg, W. S. and Smith, A. N. (1953). Release of histamine by tryptamine and 5-hydroxytryptamine. *Brit. J. Pharmacol.* **8**, 406.

Feldstein, A., Hoagland, H., Freeman, H. and Williamson, O. (1967). The effect of ethanol ingestion on serotonin–C^{14} metabolism in man. *Life Sci.* **6**, 53.

Freedland, R. A., Wadzinski, I. M. and Waisman, H. A. (1961). The enzymatic hydroxylation of tryptophan. *Biochem. Biophys. Res. Commun.* **5**, 94.

Garattini, S. and Valzelli, L. (1965). Serotonin. Elsevier, Amsterdam.

Grahame-Smith, D. G. (1967a). The biosynthesis of 5-hydroxytryptamine in carcinoid tumours and intestine. *Clin. Sci.* **33**, 147.

Grahame-Smith, D. G. (1967b). The biosynthesis of 5-hydroxytryptamine in brain. *Biochem. J.* **105**, 351.

Grahame-Smith, D. G. (1964). Tryptophan hydroxylation in carcinoid tumours. *Biochim. piophys. Acta,* **86**, 1964.

Granérus, G., Lindell, S. E., Waldenström, J., Westling, H. and White, T. (1966). Histamine metabolism in carcinoidosis. *Lancet,* **1**, 1267.

Gowenlock, A. H. and Platt, D. S. (1962). *The Clinical Chemistry of Carcinoid Tumours in the Clinical Chemistry of Monoamines* (eds H. Varley and A. H. Gowenlock), Vol. 2, p. 140. Elsevier, New York.

Gowenlock, A. H., Platt, D. S., Campbell, A. C. P. and Wormsley, K. G. (1964). Oat cell carcinoma of the bronchus secreting 5-hydroxytryptophan. *Lancet,* **1**, 304.

Jacobson, W. and Simpson, D. M. (1946). The fluorescence spectra of pterins and their possible use in the elucidation of the antipernicious anaemia factor. *Pt. 2. Biochem. J.,* **40**, 9.

Hagen, P. (1962). Observations on the substrate specificity of DOPA decarboxylase from ox adrenal medulla; human phaeochromocytoma and human argentaffinoma. *Brit. J. Pharmacol.* **18**, 175.

Hamlin, K. E. and Fischer, F. E. (1951). The synthesis of 5-hydroxytryptamine. *J. Am. Chem. Soc.* **73**, 5007.

Hilton, S. M. and Lewis, G. P. (1956). The relationship between glandular activity, bradykinin formation and functional vasodilatation in the submandibular salivary gland. *J. Physiol.* **134**, 471.

Kahlson, G., Rosengren, E., Svahn, D. and Thunberg, R. (1964). Mobilisation and formation of histamine in the gastric mucosa as related to acid secretion. *J. Physiol.* **174**, 400.

Koe, B. K. and Weissman, A. (1966). p-Chlorophenylalanine: specific depletor of brain serotonin. *J. Pharmacol. and Exper. Therap.* **154**, 499.

Langemann, V. H. *Amino Acid Decarboxylase and Amino Oxidase in Carcinoid Tumour. 5-hydroxytryptamine* (ed. G. P. Lewis), p. 159. Macmillan (Pergamon), New York.

Levine, R. J. and Sjoerdsma, A. (1963). Pressor amines and the carcinoid flush. *Ann. Int. Med.* **58**, 818.

Lewis, G. P. (1968). Kinins. *J. Roy. Coll. Phycns. Lond.* **2**, 353.

Lovenberg, W., Weissbach, H. and Udenfriend, S. (1962). Aromatic L-amine and decarboxylase. *J. Biol. Chem.* **237**, 89.

Lovenberg, W., Jequier, E. and Sjoerdsma, A. (1967). Tryptophan hydroxylation: Measurement in pineal gland, brain stem and carcinoid tumour. *Science* **155**, 217.

Lovenberg, W., Weissbach, H. and Udenfriend, S. (1962). Aromatic L-amino acid decarboxylase. *J. Biol. Chem.* **237**, 89.

McIssac, W. M. and Page, I. H. (1959). The metabolism of serotonin (5-hydroxytryptamine). *J. Biol. Chem.* **234**, 858.

Melmon, K., Lovenberg, W. and Sjoerdsma, A. (1965). Identification of· lysylbradykinin as the peptide formed *in vitro* by carcinoid tymour kallikrein. *Clin. Chem. Acta,* **12**, 292.

Mitoma, C., Posner, H. S., Roits, H. C. and Udenfriend, S. (1956). Enzymatic hydroxylation of aromatic compounds. *Arch. Biochem. Biophys.* **61**, 431.

Oates, J. A. and Sjoerdsma, A. (1962). A unique syndrome associated with secretion of 5-hydroxytryptophan by metastatic gastric carcinoids. *Am. J. Med.* **32**, 333.

Oates, J. A., Melmon, K., Sjoerdsma, A., Gillespie, L. and Mason, D. T. (1964). Release of a kinin peptide in the carcinoid syndrome. *Lancet*, **1**, 514.

Oates, J. A. and Sjoerdsma, A. (1962). A unique syndrome associated with secreting of 5-hydroxytryptophan by metastatic gastric carcinoids. *Am. J. Med.* **32**, 333.

O'Connor, J. M. (1912). Uber der Adrenalingehalt des Blutes. *Arch. Exper. Path. v. Pharmacol.* **67**, 195.

Page, I. H., Corcoran, A. C., Udenfriend, S., Sjoerdsma, A. and Weissbach, H. (1955). Argentaffinoma as an endocrine tumour. *Lancet*, **1**, 198.

Pernow, B. and Waldenström, J. (1957). Determination of 5-hydroxytryptamine, 5-hydroxyindole acetic acid and histamine in thirty three cases of carcinoid tumours (argentaffinoma). *Am. J. Med.* **23**, 16.

Prusoff, W. H. (1960). The distribution of 5-hydroxytryptamine and adenosin triphosphate in cytoplasmic particles of the dog's small intestine. *Brit. J. Pharmacol.* **15**, 520.

Rapport, M. M. (1949). Serum vasoconstrictor (serotonin) V. The presence of creatinine in the complex. A proposed structure of the vasoconstrictor principle. *J. Biol. Chem.* **180**, 961.

Rapport, M. M., Green, A. A. and Page, I. H. (1948). Serum vasoconstrictor (serotonin) IV. Isolation and characterisation. *J. Biol. Chem.* **176**, 1243.

Renson, J., Weissbach, H. and Udenfriend, S. (1962). The hydroxylation of tryptophan by phenylalanine hydroxylase. *J. Biol. Chem.* **237**, 2261.

Robertson, J. I. S., Peart, W. S. and Andrews, T. M. (1962). The mechanism of facial flushes in the carcinoid syndrome. *Quart. J. Med.* **21**, 103.

Sauer, W. G., Dearing, W. H., Flock, E. V., Waugh, J. M., Dockerty, M. E. and Roth, G. M. (1958). Functioning carcinoid tumours. *Gastroenterology.* **34**, 216.

Sandler, M. and Snow, P. D. J. (1958). An atypical carcinoid tumour secreting 5-hydroxytryptophan. *Lancet*, **1**, 137.

Schindler, R. (1958). The conversion of ^{14}C labelled tryptophan to 5-hydroxytryptamine by neoplastic mast cells. *Biochem. Pharmacol.* **1**, 323.

Sjoerdsma, A., Weissbach, H. and Udenfriend, S. (1956). A clinical, physiologic and biochemical study of patients with malignant carcinoid (argentaffinoma). *Am. J. Med.* **20**, 520.

Sjoerdsma, A., Weissbach, H., Terry, L. L. and Udenfriend, S. (1957). Further observations on patients with malignant carcinoid. *Am. J. Med.* **23**, 5.

Smith, A. N., Nyhus, L. M., Dalgleish, C. E., Dutton, R. W., Lennox, B. and MacFarlane, P. S. (1957). Further observations on the endocrine aspects of argentaffinoma. *Scot. Med. J.* **2**, 24.

Titus, E. and Udenfriend, S. (1954). Metabolism of 5-hydroxytryptamine (Serotonin). *Fed. Proc.* **13**, 411.

Udenfriend, S., Titus, E., Weissbach, H. and Peterson, R. E. (1956). Biogenesis and metabolism of 5-hydroxyindole compounds. *J. Biol. Chem.* **219**, 335.

Udenfriend, S., Creveling, C. R., Posner, H., Redfield, B. G., Daly, J. and Witkop, B. (1959). On the inability of tryptamine to serve as a precursor of serotonin. *Arch. Biochem. Biophys.* **83**, 501.

Udenfriend, S., Clark, C. T. and Titus, E. (1953). Hydroxylation of the 5-position of tryptophan as the first step in its metabolic conversion to 5-hydroxytryptamine (serotonin). *Fed. Proc.* **12**, 282.

Vane, J. R. (1969). Release and fate of vasoactive hormones in the circulation. *Brit. J. Pharmacol.* **35**, 209.

Waldenström, J. and Ljungberg, E. (1956). Case of metastasing carcinoma of unknown origin showing peculiar red flushing and increased amounts of histamine and 5-hydroxytryptamine on blood and urine. *Acta Med. Scand.* **153**, 73.

Weissbach, H., Redfield, B. G. and Udenfriend, S. (1957). Soluble monoamine oxidase; its properties and action on serotonin. *J. Biol. Chem.* **229**, 953.

Zeitlhofer, J. and Formanek, K. (1959). Beitrag zum sogenannten Carcinoid syndrom. *Zentr. Allegm. Pathol. Anat.* **99**, 306.

CHAPTER 5

Clinical Aspects

Production of symptoms

The symptoms of the carcinoid syndrome appear to be due to either the effects of its humoral secretions or to the local effects of the tumour and its metastases. It is a matter of observation that with those tumours arising in sites, the venous drainage of which is via the portal venous system, the symptoms, such as flushing and diarrhoea which we associate with humoral secretions, do not occur until hepatic metastases are present. On the other hand, bronchial and ovarian tumours, draining their products into the systemic circulation, may produce the syndrome without metastatic spread. It has been suggested, therefore, that in the case of intestinal primaries, the liver lies between the tumour and the systemic circulation and that until hepatic metastases occur which drain their products into the systemic circulation, the liver acts to inactivate the tumour's humoral products. On the whole this is the most reasonable suggestion. The alternative explanation is that usually the primary intestinal tumour is small and remains small and that hepatic metastases allow the growth of a sufficient mass of tumour to produce the quantities of humoral products necessary to produce symptoms. Unfortunately, all this means that by the time the carcinoid syndrome results in patients with gastrointestinal primaries there is already hepatic metastatic spread.

The clinical manifestations of the carcinoid syndrome and their pharmacological and biochemical basis

From the first reports in the early 1950's it became apparent quickly that the cardinal manifestations of the disease were flushing, diarrhoea, cardiac valvular lesions, and wheezing. In Table 8, taken from an excellent review by Thorson (1958), are shown the chief symptoms and signs with some indication of their frequency.

In my own experience flushing is the most common symptom, with diarrhoea as a close second. Cardiac valvular lesions come next but

41

TABLE 8

The incidence of manifestations of the carcinoid syndrome (from Thorson, 1958)

Total number of cases*	79
Male 48	
Female 29	
Age at presentation	
Male	18-80
Female	33-80
Flushing	74
Intestinal hypermotility	68
Asthma	18
Edema	52
Heart lesions	41
Pellagra-like skin lesions	5
Peptic ulcers	5
Arthralgia	6

* The sex of 2 patients is not reported in the literature.

wheezing of any significant degree I have only seen in five cases out of about 40. Other manifestations occur sporadically. Nevertheless, the combination and differing quality of these major features and their coupling with the less common symptoms and signs make up the syndrome which has subtle variations from patient to patient and composes the 'Carcinoid Spectrum'. I suspect that these differences reflect most probably the capacity of the tumour to produce different quantities and types of hormones and the patient's individual reaction to them.

Occurrence

With lack of information 'Epidemiology' would be a too pretentious term to describe this aspect. The general incidence, geographical and spcial incidence of the carcinoid syndrome is unknown. One cannot simply equate this with the evidence of carcinoid tumours, which are relatively common. Linell and Månsson (1966), discussing the overall prevalence and incidence of carcinoids in Malmo, Sweden, make the statement, 'As a rough guess it (*the carcinoid syndrome*) might occur once or twice every ten years in the population of Malmo (230,000 inhabitants)'. At St Mary's Hospital over the past ten years I have seen 40 cases with the proven syndrome. All but two of these cases have been referred from other hospitals and this number is only reflection of a personal interest.

There appears to be no sex difference in incidence and the age of presentation varies greatly from 18 to 76 years in my own patients. The time of presentation of the syndrome may be many years after the occurrence of the tumour. In one patient a primary ileal tumour was removed in 1957 because of abdominal pain. The carcinoid syndrome with multiple hepatic metastases did not present until 1969, i.e. twelve years later. Frequently, from observation of the growth of the tumour and its metastases, one suspects the tumour must have been present many years before the patient presents with symptoms of the syndrome.

Sandler (1968) has raised the possibility that there may be a predisposition to the carcinoid tumour and its syndrome. This is an interesting proposition but what is the evidence? He refers to a number of reports in which flushing had been present since early life. Funk *et al.* (1966) made the interesting observation that in non-carcinoid patients with renal cysts there was an increase in the number of gastrointestinal argentaffin cells, perhaps linking some aspect of renal function with a trophic effect upon argentaffin cells. Neither of these observations are very impressive but the common occurrence of multiple carcinoid primaries and the occasional striking case such as that described by Black and Haffner (1968) in which hundreds of small gastric carcinoids were present together with an excess of argyrophilic cells in the stomach are impressive. Hedinger (1966) found no important increase in the overall number of argentaffin cells in 12 patients with the carcinoid syndrome, though one-third had renal cysts compared with one-ninth of a control autopsy group. There is also the association of the carcinoid syndrome with the pluriglandular adenomas to be considered (Williams and Celestin, 1962). These facts raise the question as to whether there is some factor controlling the growth and function of enterochromaffin cells and whether the growth of carcinoid tumours could be initiated or maintained from some unknown source.

Flushing

Of all the manifestations of the carcinoid syndrome the flushing shows the greatest variation, a knowledge of which can be of help in the clinical assessment of the individual case. I have previously subdivided flushing into four types (Grahame-Smith, 1968).

1. A diffuse erythematous flush usually affecting mainly the face, neck and upper anterior chest (i.e. the normal flushing area) but on close observation often being more widespread and visibly affecting the skin of the back and abdomen and palms. This type of flush is most frequently paroxysmal and commonly shortlived, lasting 2-5 min. Quite often this type of flush occurs in patients with a normal 'non-flushing' colour to their face.

2. This flush has a violaceous tinge to it. It affects the same areas but lasts a little longer than type 1. The nose is often a shining purple beacon during a flush, which tends to occur on a background of a permanent cyanotic flush. Such patients often show dilated facial veins and telangiectases, suffused conjunctivae and watery eyes.

3. This type of flush is most commonly associated with bronchial carcinoid tumours. The flushes often last several hours and may even last 2-3 days. The skin, particularly in the flushing areas, becomes red but not so startling a red as in type 1. Other body areas are frequently involved. There is profuse lacrimation and the conjunctivae are red. Palpitations associated with increased cardiac output are sometimes present. The facial skin swells and the normal facial creases become exaggerated into deep folds. Hypotension may be present and the salivary glands often swell. Patients often have exacerbation of diarrhoea concurrently. This type of flushing is the most physically distressing.

4. This is a bright red but patchy flush, the red flush appearing a particularly vivid red and the white patches appearing a particularly bright white. This patchiness for some reason is often seen around the root of the neck. This type of flushing seems to be associated with gastric carcinoid tumours and an excess histamine production.

I believe these four types of flushing are distinct. Elsewhere I have argued (Grahame-Smith, 1968) that perhaps type 1 is a forerunner of type 2, but I am beginning to doubt this. I have observed two patients now with type 1 flushing over the last six years and although there is no doubt that their faces show a general increase in colour, particularly on the forehead, cheeks and nose, there is no real permanent cyanotic tinge to this colour such as one sees in type 3. Backing evidence for this view is the fact that in those who are cyanotic and have cyanotic flushes one does not get a history of preceding erythematous flushing of type 1. It suggests that the pharmacology of these different types of flushing is dissimilar.

Many everyday things tend to precipitate carcinoid flushing. Certain foods, such as cheese and salty bacon, may be responsible. More common is a simple relationship to meal times, particularly noticeable is the flushing occurring after the first hot drink of the day. Alcohol in any form is often a potent provocation of flushing. One of my patients first noticed flushing one Christmas when he ate Christmas pudding with rum sauce. Some patients notice flushing only with the first alcoholic drink of a sequence. After that, and for some hours, alcohol has no effect. The pharmacological basis of these reactions is discussed on pages 45-54. Excitement also provokes flushing and here circulating adrenaline may be the trigger as it may well be for exertion. One of our patients had his first and overwhelming flush when trying to keep upright a small boat in which he and his family were out at sea during a swell.

The pattern of flushing and factors which precipitate it are not only of interest but also of diagnostic importance. Many older women present with the carcinoid syndrome complaining of a return of menopausal flushing. My own observations of menopausal flushing I should like to record here. The menopausal hot flush (or 'flash' in the U.S.A.) differs from the carcinoid flush. First there is often very little flushing, the patient feeling hot, sweaty and uncomfortable, but not going very red, if at all. Rarely in menopausal flushing does one get a good history of precipitating factors and they seem to last longer than carcinoid flushes, which incidentally are rarely accompanied by much sweating. Menopausal sensations are not precipitated by I.V. catecholamine, and the sensations women experience during the menopausal flush are quite different from those experienced in a carcinoid flush.

The severity of carcinoid flushing is very variable. It can vary from transient, hardly visible reddening, to more prolonged beetroot colouring. Flushing on a violaceous background can sometimes be difficult to detect, though in those cases there is plainly a potent and continuous stimulus to vasodilatation. In several patients severe flushing has been observed to be followed by prominence of peripheral veins in the forearm and whiteness of the skin over and on either side of the veins. In other patients during the dying phase of a flush, patchy clearing occurs. Some patients feel generally unwell during a flush (type 1 and 2) but on the whole, apart from the embarrassment, mild flushing is not disabling.

Type 3 flushing on the other hand is disabling and bronchial carcinoid patients with this type of flushing may benefit from treatment with glucocorticoid steroid derivatives which frequently suppress this type of flush. For example, two patients with metastatic bronchial tumours have flushed for days at a time. During a flush, involving total body surface, the whole face swelled, the eyes watered, entropion occurred, salivary glands swelled, hypotension with tachycardia and forceful cardiac pulsations which kept them awake were present. The haemodynamic consequences of this type of flushing are discussed on page 54. Clearly, this type of flushing is in a different category.

One point of interest, for which there is no explanation, is that many patients say that the flush seems to start with a sensation in the epigastrium and that the sensation spreads upwards over the anterior chest wall to appear in the face and neck as a flush. Could the sensation in the epigastrium be due to the release of kallikrein from hepatic metastases?

Biochemical Pharmacology of Flushing

Until 1960 it was widely accepted that the carcinoid flush was due to the paroxysmal release of 5HT into the circulation, indeed Page and

McCubbin (1953) reported that I.V. 5HT would cause facial flushing in both normal and carcinoid patients. However, certain factors were against 5HT causing the carcinoid flush.

1. Flushing might be severe in patients with little increase in urinary 5HIAA. In other cases there might be very little flushing with large increases in urinary 5HIAA.
2. Robertson *et al.* (1962) showed that when 5HT was given I.V. to carcinoid patients that overbreathing, tingling around the mouth and nose, transient but sometimes severe headache, occurred at doses necessary to cause a rather uninmpressive cyanotic flush and that in these same patients with the carcinoid syndrome their spontaneous or catecholamine-induced flushing was not accompanied by these other symptoms. In addition, several patients had a rise in blood pressure during the mild flush produced by 5HT, a feature not noted in their natural flushes.
3. Robertson *et al.* (1962) also measured the concentration of 5HT free in the plasma. One of the problems in measuring blood 5HT is that the majority is bound to platelets and is presumably unavailable for pharmacological activity, while the unbound 5HT, free in the plasma, is of very low concentration. The technical difficulties in separating

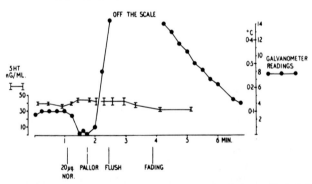

Fig. 5. Absence of a rise of free plasma serotonin during a flush induced by intravenous noradrenaline in a patient with the carcinoid syndrome. A flush was induced by the injection of 20 micrograms of noradrenaline intravenously. It was preceded by the usual facial pallor. The trace indicated by • represents galvanometer readings of skin temperature detected by a heat-sensitive disc. During the noradrenaline-induced flush blood was taken from an indwelling catheter in the upper inferior vena cava and the content of samples of blood withdrawn during the flush were assayed for 5HT by a bioassay method. As shown above, no rise in the free plasma 5HT concentration was found during the flush.

off blood platelets ensuring that no 5HT is released artefactually are considerable and perhaps our knowledge of the true level of free plasma 5HT is faulty. Despite these constraints, Robertson and his colleagues were unable to find any rise in the level of free plasma 5HT during a flush, in the majority of the patients they studied (Fig. 5), despite the fact that the 5HT in the plasma of superior vena caval blood rose after the injection of 5HT into an ankle vein in amounts insufficient to cause flushing (Fig. 6). In one patient, however, flushing was accompanied by a rise in free plasma 5HT and in this patient the flush was of a cyanotic type and was accompanied by hyperventilation (Fig. 7). Thus, although 5HT may be involved in some patients it was clearly not the major factor causing the flush.

RECOVERY OF SEROTONIN FROM RIGHT ATRIAL PLASMA.
SEROTONIN INJECTION INTO ANKLE VEIN.

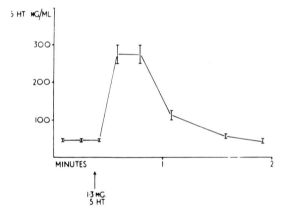

Fig. 6. The rise of free plasma serotonin after the intravenous injection of serotonin. As shown above, when 1.3 mg of serotonin was injected into an ankle vein the free plasma serotonin in the right atrial blood increased considerably but fell back to normal levels after two minutes. This injection was not accompanied by flushing and shows that the experiment depicted in Fig. 5 was, in its negative sense, valid.

The next step was taken by Oates *et al.* (1964). Searching for another vasodilating agent and noting that catecholamines which provoke carcinoid flushing also provoke an increase of bradykinin secretion within the salivary gland, they studied the role which bradykinin might have in the carcinoid flush.

Briefly, their findings were:

1. Bradykinin caused flushing, tachycardia and hypotension in their patients (though hypotension has not been a common feature of

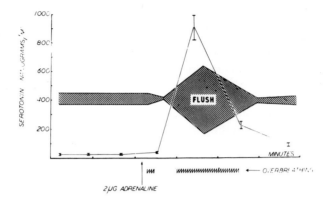

Fig. 7. In one patient who had a pancreatic adenocarcinoma associated with the carcinoid syndrome and cyanotic flushing accompanied by overbreathing (Peart *et al.*, 1963) flushing was found to be accompanied by a rise of free plasma serotonin, as shown above. After an intravenous injection of 2 micrograms of adrenaline there was short episode of overbreathing due to the direct effect of adrenaline, after which a flush quickly appeared which was accompanied by a rise in the free plasma serotonin level.

flushing in my patients). These effects were reproduced in spontaneous or catecholamine-provoked flushing.

2. Bradykinin levels in hepatic venous blood draining liver metastases rose considerably during provoked flushing.

3. That the tumour contained a glandular kallikrein which when incubated with human kininogen produced lysyl-bradykinin, which is converted to bradykinin by plasma amino peptidase (Melmon, Lovenberg and Sjoerdsma, 1965).

These results have been broadly confirmed by Zeitlin and Smith, 1966; Oates *et al.*, 1966; and Adamson *et al.*, 1968. On the face of it, bradykinin seems to be a real factor in the production of flushing, though it is necessary always to keep in mind that it is the enzyme kallikrein which is the functional secretion from the tumour. However, there are objections to bradykinin being the only flush producing factor:

First, not in all patients can a rise in plasma bradykinin be demonstrated (Oates *et al.*, 1966; Adamson *et al.*, 1968). Secondly, there is no doubt that intravenous bradykinin, in most carcinoid patients, does not reproduce exactly a flush which is a qualitative replica of their spontaneous flush. The main features which are different are that the bradykinin flush is much pinker than the spontaneous flush, and that tachycardia and hypotension are in my experience more marked. Bradykinin does not produce much hyperventilation, cyanosis or any of the patchy skin discoloration often seen in carcinoid flushing. Possibly 5HT might be acting synergistically, causing venous constriction and stagnant anoxia (and therefore cyanosis) of blood contained with the arterioles dilated by bradykinin.

Because bradykinin is not the whole story the hunt for vasodilating materials has continued. Sandler, Karim and Williams (1968) have discovered that some bronchial carcinoid tumours contain a prostaglandin and ileal carcinoids an unknown hydroxy-fatty acid which may be a prostaglandin. Since prostaglandins have widespread pharmacological effects, including vasodilatation, their production by carcinoid tumours needs further exploration. In addition, a new vasodilating polypeptide has been discovered in intestinal mucosa by Said and Mutt (1970) and the role of this in the carcinoid syndrome should be investigated.

The matter of flush provocation is of general pharmacological interest. Schneckloth *et al.* (1957) and Stacey (1957) reported that noradrenaline and adrenaline would provoke carcinoid flushing. Peart, Andrews and Robertson (1959) studied this in greater detail and Levine and Sjoerdsma (1963) studied the potency of a range of catecholamines and related substances in provoking flushing (for example see Table 9).

TABLE 9

Relative potency of vasoactive amines in causing carcinoid flushing
(from Levine and Sjoerdsma, 1963)

Amine	Dose μg	Flush
Adrenaline	0.6-5	++++
Isoprenaline	1-10	++++
Noradrenaline	1-10	++++
Tyramine	500-750	++ to ++++
Meteraminol	500-2000	+ to ++
Mephentermine	1000-2000	0 to ++
Methoxamine	4000-10,000	0 to +

Recently, my colleagues and I have been interested in the mechanisms by which catecholamines and alcohol cause the release of flush producing substances from the tumour. These investigations are worth relating in some detail because the findings form a background for the flush provocation test described on page 69, and also give some insight into the pharmacology of secretion of kallikrein by the neoplastic enterochromaffin cell. On the assumption that flushing associated with a rise in arterial plasma-bradykinin reflects the paroxysmal release of kallikrein from the tumour, we studied the factors controlling this release in patients with the carcinoid syndrome.

In a typical case (Fig. 8) I.V. bradykinin (60 μg) caused flushing within 40 s, the flush lasting about 50 s, and the flush was not preceded by any observable effect. Twenty seconds after noradrenaline I.V. (6 μg) hyperventilation occurred and was accompanied by facial pallor. Hyperventilation lasted about 10 s and pallor 15-20 s. These are expected pharmacological effects of noradrenaline occurring within the circulation time. Seventy-five seconds after noradrenaline the flush began. Figure 9 shows the blood bradykinin level at the height of the flush when bradykinin and noradrenaline respectively are given. The flushing obtained with bradykinin is due to an immediate effect of bradykinin on the blood vessels and is not dependent upon intermediate events such as the release of tumour kallikrein. On the other hand, it is probable that noradrenaline circulated to the tumour, during which time pallor and hyperventilation occur, that noradrenaline stimulates the release of kallikrein and that by the action of kallikrein, the bradykinin

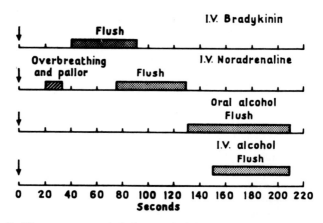

Fig. 8. Time sequence of flush provoked by oral and intravenous alcohol compared with that of intravenous bradykinin and intravenous noradrenaline. In a patient with a metastatic ileal carcinoid tumour. The administration of each substance is indicated by the arrow at zero time. Note that the flush precipitated by intravenous bradykinin, 60 μg, came on at about 40 s and disappeared at about 90 s. The flush response to intravenous noradrenaline was preceded by a short period within the circulation of time of overbreathing and pallor. The flush with noradrenaline did not occur until about 70 s and lasted until about 130 s. With alcohol, 4 ml of 95% alcohol in 10 ml of orange juice, the flush did not occur until 130 s and was over at 210 s. The flush induced by 10 ml of alcohol (4.75%) given intravenously came on and disappeared with roughly the same time sequence as that induced by oral alcohol.

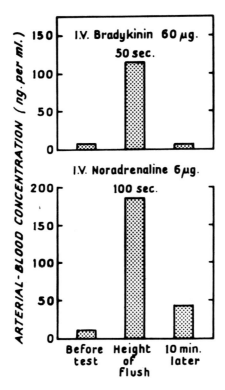

Fig. 9. Arterial blood bradykinin concentrations during flush provoked by intravenous bradykinin and intravenous noradrenaline. After intravenous bradykinin, at the height of the flush, bradykinin was measurable in the arterial blood by a bioassay technique. Below is shown the rise in arterial blood bradykinin at the height of a flush induced by intravenous noradrenaline.

concentration of the blood is raised to flushing levels and this sequence takes time. Noradrenaline-induced flushing was blocked by intravenous phentolamine or by oral phenoxybenzamine (α-adrenergic blocking agents) in all seven patients studied. Bradykinin-induced flushing was not so blocked. When noradrenaline-induced flushing was blocked there was no rise in the plasma bradykinin level after I.V. noradrenaline (see Fig. 10).

In some patients (5 out of 12) flushing occurred in response to oral alcohol (e.g. 4 ml 95% ethanol in 10 ml orange juice). In contrast to both bradykinin and noradrenaline, alcohol-induced flushing was delayed, the flush beginning at 130-150 s after ingestion (see Fig. 7). I.V. alcohol (10 ml of 4.75% solution) produced flushing with the same time sequence. Not all patients were responsive to alcohol and some who

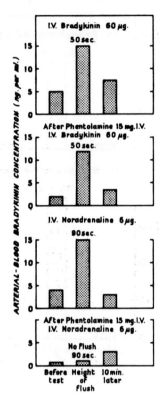

Fig. 10. Phentolamine blockade of the rise in bradykinin concentrations after intravenous noradrenaline but not that after intravenous bradykinin. In the upper two sections of this figure are shown first, the effect of intravenous bradykinin to cause a rise during flushing of the blood bradykinin concentration and below that, the lack of effect of phentolamine upon either the flushing or the rise in intravenous bradykinin. The upper of the lower two sections shows the rise of arterial blood bradykinin in this patient with the carcinoid syndrome after an injection of intravenous noradrenaline, and below that, the effect of phentolamine to block both the flush and the rise in blood bradykinin.

were, did not respond to a further dose of alcohol given soon after the first and required several hours to recover their responsiveness. They did, however, respond to both noradrenaline and bradykinin during this period so that their flushing potential was unimpaired. Alcohol-induced flushing was also accompanied by a rise in the plasma bradykinin level (Fig. 10). When unresponsive to alcohol, there was no rise in plasma bradykinin. Surprisingly, alcohol-induced flushing was blocked in two patients by I.V. phentolamine.

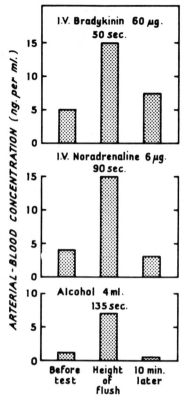

Fig. 11. Arterial blood bradykinin concentrations during a flush provoked by intravenous bradykinin, intravenous noradrenaline and oral alcohol. Again the rise in blood bradykinin levels induced by intravenous bradykinin and by intravenous noradrenaline is compared with the rise in blood bradykinin levels induced by oral alcohol during a flush. There is no doubt that alcohol causes a release of kallikrein from the tumour and the subsequent increase in the blood bradykinin levels.

We have suggested that alcohol acts to release an endogenous catecholamine which circulates to the tumour to release kallikrein. The release of this catecholamine and the unresponsiveness in some patients to a second dose of alcohol could be brought about by a depletion of this catecholamine store. Dopamine and noradrenaline are unlikely candidates for the identity of this catecholamine since the action of these amines can be blocked by α-adrenergic blocking agents while alcohol-induced flushing is still present. Adrenaline is unlikely because there is no evidence such as pallor or hyperventilation of a sudden release of adrenaline into the circulation. Further studies are necessary to elucidate entirely these interesting effects of alcohol.

At no time were we able to block catecholamine-induced flushing with the β-adrenergic blocking agent propranolol, even though the lipolytic and chronotropic effects of adrenaline were blocked. Oates and Butler (1967) have also failed to block catecholamine-induced flushing with propranolol.

The mechanism of catecholamine-induced release of kallikrein is not understood but catecholamines and sympathetic stimulation do release kallikrein from salivary gland (Hilton and Lewis, 1956) so that these effects are involved in normal tissues as well as in the carcinoid tumour.

Occasionally during flushing severe headache is experienced. This could be due to histamine or prostaglandins, both of these substances causing headache when given intravenously.

In one patient with severe, type 3, flushing there occurred during the flush severe palpitations which shook the bed. The pulse was regular and of extremely high amplitude and the precordial pulsation increased greatly during a flush. Cardiac output rose from a non-flushing level of 5.75 L/min to a flushing level of 7.98 L/min and the femoral artery blood flow from 644 cc/min to 1250 cc/min. The increase in cardiac output and limb blood flow is, therefore, quite marked during flushing.

Diarrhoea

While flushing is in my experience the most common symptom this is followed a close second by diarrhoea. Some patients may have no diarrhoea, only flushing; others note the passage of one or two watery stools per day, usually accompanied by some urgency of defaecation. Others have severe diarrhoea with the frequent passage of unformed watery stools accompanied by abdominal cramping pains, borborygmi and explosive defaecation. The diarrhoea may or may not bear a temporal or quantitative relationship to the flushing but the striking dissociation in many patients forces one to conclude that flushing and diarrhoea are not due to the same humoral secretion. Occasionally it seems that diarrhoea is due to a local effect of the tumour on the gastrointestinal tract but this is unusual. On some occasions, and this cannot be ignored, the flushing and diarrhoea are temporally related and in these cases it would seem that both the flush and diarrhoea promoting hormones are being secreted together. Removal of tumour metastases by hepatic resection has completely cured the diarrhoea in three of our cases, and the diarrhoea has also been cured by the removal of a non-metastatic non-gastrointestinal tumour (Waldenström, 1958).

If these facts point to a humoral cause for diarrhoea what is its nature? Most interest has focused on 5HT in this regard. 5HT is normally found in gastrointestinal mucosa (Feldberg and Toh, 1953) and more recently Bulbring and Gershon (1967) have shown that 5HT is also synthesized and stored in nerve endings in the myenteric plexus, to be released on stimulation of preganglionic nerves. it would seem that in the normal gut there are two functional stores of 5HT and the precise role of each of these in the maintenance of normal intestinal activity is not clear.

Although the mucosal store of 5HT can be greatly depleted by a tryptophan deficient state (Boullin, 1964) and peristalsis remains unaffected it could be that enough 5HT remains for normal function. Certainly 5HT is released into the venous effluent of normal intestine when the intestine is stimulated by scratching of the serosal surface, intra-arterial acetylcholine and increased intraluminal pressure (Burks and Long, 1966). On the one hand there is the suggestion that 5HT has neurohumoral actions in the myenteric plexus of the gut (Bulbring and Gershon, 1967) and on the other that 5HT may alter the threshold of excitation of mucosal sensory nerve endings so that a lower pressure in the intestine is required to elicit the peristaltic reflex (Page, 1968). Further work will no doubt unravel the problem of the role of 5HT in the maintenance of intestinal motor activity.

More relevant to the carcinoid syndrome are the observations on the action of 5HT upon human intestinal mobility. 5HT directly stimulates the small gut and inhibits the large (Bennett and Whitney, 1966; Fishlock and Parks, 1966; Hendrix *et al.*, 1957). Misiewicz *et al.* (1966) have also shown that *in vivo* 5HT stimulates the small intestine and inhibits the mobility of the stomach and colon. One could explain diarrhoea on this basis by assuming that the intestinal contents expelled into the colon by a hypermotile small gut pass quickly through an immotile colon into the rectum to initiate a defaecation reflex. Misiewicz *et al.* (1966) have shown that the pattern of intestinal motility induced by 5HT is not unlike that seen in the carcinoid syndrome. The difficulties as I see them in this interpretation are:

1. Paroxysmal rises in free plasma 5HT levels are unusual in the carcinoid syndrome.
2. Both bradykinin and prostaglandins have actions upon gut motility which confuse the clinical picture.

It would be of interest to examine the intestinal wall content of 5HT in the carcinoid syndrome to see whether the mucosal stores of 5HT are increased by uptake from the increased blood concentration.

There is some indirect evidence that 5HT may be responsible for the diarrhoea. First, 5HT pharmacological antagonists such as methysergide are often extremely effective in combating the diarrhoea (though the specificity of pharmacological antagonists is always a matter of doubt). Second, p-chlorophenylalanine is sometimes effective in controlling the diarrhoea and this prevents the synthesis of 5HT (Engleman, Lovenberg and Sjoerdsma, 1967).

Malabsorption in the carcinoid syndrome

Malabsorption is an unusual manifestation of the carcinoid syndrome but has been reported (Kowlessar *et al.,* 1959; Nash and Brin, 1964; Melmon *et al.,* 1963). Faecal fat excretion of greater than 75 G/day have been found. In the patients studied by Melmon *et al.* (1963) biopsy of the jejunal mucosa revealed no abnormalities, and although previous ileal resection is sometimes a possible cause this does not seem to be the major factor. Lymphatic obstruction by tumour or fibrosis might theoretically be causative. However, there is striking improvement of the malabsorption when methysergide is given, suggesting that 5HT in some way is involved (Melmon *et al.,* 1963). If diarrhoea alone were the cause, then all carcinoid patients with severe diarrhoea would be expected to have a major degree of malabsorption and this is not the case. Elevation of urinary 5HIAA has been noted in the adult coeliac syndrome (Haverback and Davidson, 1958; Kowlessar *et al.,* 1958). The meaning of this is not clear and the role of 5HT in intestinal absorptive processes has not been defined. Nevertheless, malabsorption should be considered in all cases of the carcinoid syndrome, particularly in relation to the cachexia which sometimes ensues and also as another factor perhaps involved in the production of pellagra.

Abdominal pain

Patients with the carcinoid syndrome frequently complain of abdominal pain and the differential diagnosis can be a difficult one. Among the causes are:
1. Peptic ulceration.
2. Intestinal obstruction due to intestinal stenosis due to tumour or associated fibrosis.
3. Pain arising from hepatic metastases.
4. Pain associated with increased intestinal motility and diarrhoea.
5. Pain arising from intestinal necrosis.

Peptic ucleration in the carcinoid syndrome has been reported by MacDonald (1956). However, it is difficult to be sure that this is a real clinical association and I have not seen it. Intestinal obstruction, however, is a real occurrence. It can arise from the primary ileal tumour and though these are usually small and not large enough to cause obstruction, on occasions they can grow large enough to cause a stricture. More commonly there is a fibrotic reaction in the region of the tumour which contributes to the stricture. The comment has been made that the intestinal muscle in the region of a carcinoid tumour is often hypertrophied (Sokoloff, 1968). More common than this is the situation which occurs after the removal by intestinal resection of a primary ileal tumour. The patient presents a year or more after this complaining of some colicky pain and on examination there is a large mass in the right iliac fossa. At laparotomy a fibrotic mass involving loops of gut is found in the region of the previous anastomosis and in this mass small clusters of argentaffin cells are present.

Pain arising from hepatic metastases is also very common. The surface of the liver which, of course, is often grossly enlarged, is usually tender over a small area and over a period of weeks the pain and tenderness disappears. During this time the symptoms of either flushing or diarrhoea increase and wane as the pain disappears. These episodes are probably due to tumour necrosis. The central portions of large hepatic metastases frequently necrose and liquefy and general malaise and worsening of the symptoms are usually associated. During these episodes the urine may contain an even greater excess of 5-hydroxyindole metabolites and some atypical to the individual patient. The diagnosis of a necrosing hepatic metastasis can usually be made on clinical grounds, and if localized by physical examination then this localization can be matched with that on a hepatic scan. Abdominal pain is most usual from hepatic metastases but I have seen pleuritic pain, right basal pleural effusion and basal bronchopneumonia due to necrosis of a large metastases beneath the right dome of the diaphragm. Some of these metastases may necrose right through the liver capsule and their contents be released into the intra-abdominal cavity. It is not surprising that when such potent pain-producing substances and irritants as 5HT and bradykinin come into contact with the peritoneum that pain should result.

The pain arising from increased intestinal motility is sometimes seen in those patients in whom flushing is associated with increased intestinal motility and borborygmi. Robertson *et al.* (1962) remark on three of their patients who experienced abdominal pain and hyperperistalsis during flushing provoked by I.V. adrenaline. Lastly, necrosis of the small intestine may be produced by infarction secondary to obstruction of mesenteric vessels by clumps of enlarged metastatic mesenteric lymph nodes.

Respiratory symptoms

From the earliest descriptions of the carcinoid syndrome 'Asthma' has been noted. Mattingly and Sjoerdsma (1956) noted asthma and respiratory distress in about 20% of their cases. The incidence has been less than this, about 10%, in the cases I have seen.

There are at least two aspects to respiratory distress in the carcinoid syndrome. First, hyperventilation occurring during flushing. This is not uncommon and it is often more noticeable to the observer than to the patient. In patients affected the hyperventilation mounts coincident with the onset and increasing severity of a flush, to disappear usually before the flush disappears. It is possible that this is due to 5HT release, and certainly in one case reported by Robertson *et al.* (1962) the hyperventilation was accompanied by a rise in the free plasma level of 5HT and intravenous injections of 5HT are very effective in causing hyperventilation. There is the impression, no more, that this hyperventilation is more common during these flushes which are cyanotic in type. it is probable, though not certain, that the cause is humoral, since measures which block flushing block the hyperventilation response too, without affecting the hyperventilation which occurs as a direct response to the injection of flush-provoking catecholamines.

The asthmatic component of the carcinoid syndrome is a more difficult symptom to be precise about. It is my experience that this symptom seems to occur clinically on a background of chronic bronchitis and emphysema and that there is, in patients affected, some degree of chronic airways obstruction which definitely and measurably worsens during a flush. Such wheezing is relieved by inhalation of an isoprenaline aerosol which does not precipitate flushing, and is worsened by the administration of β-adrenergic blocking agents. In one case studied by Professor C. T. Dollery there was an equivocal improvement in the wheezing associated with flushing provoked by noradrenaline when the patient was receiving methysergide. Mengel (1965) has stated that I.V. methysergide is effective in overcoming bronchoconstriction during anaesthesia, suggesting that 5HT may be responsible. Obviously adrenaline subcutaneously should never be given to relieve the asthma of the carcinoid syndrome, since this would worsen flushing and presumably release more of the humoral mediator of broncho-constriction from the tumour. While 5HT appears to be a candidate for causation of the wheezing, bradykinin and histamine are both effective in certain species in causing bronchoconstriction.

Fibrosis and the carcinoid syndrome

The occurrence of fibrosis in the heart is not the only situation when an excess of fibrous tissue is seen in the carcinoid syndrome. Peritoneal fibrosis, particularly in the pelvic region, has frequently been reported (Cassidy, 1930, 1931; Cosh *et al.,* 1959; Eder and Schauer, 1959; Fabricius *et al.,* 1958; Fadell and Denham, 1966; Hallen, 1964; Hedinger and Gloor, 1964; Olesen, 1955; Torvik, 1960). Lung adhesions (Jatlow and Rice, 1964) and constrictive pericarditis (Dockerty and Scheifley, 1955) have also been reported. In a personal case, fibrosis in the retroperitoneal region and in the pelvis involved the ureters causing obstructive renal failure and such ureteric involvement has been described (Bates and Clark, 1963; Hale and Lane-Mitchell, 1964; House and Hermann, 1965). Retroperitoneal fibrosis has also been reported after administration of methysergide, the 5HT antagonist (Carr and Biswas, 1966; Utz *et al.,* 1965; Schwartz *et al.,* 1966), the molecular structure of which contains a portion like 5HT.

Cardiac lesions

To the clinician one of the most striking features of the carcinoid syndrome is the occurrence of a specific form of heart disease. So unusual is this that it is possible in retrospect to pick out from the literature cases of the carcinoid syndrome reported prior to its general recognition (Cassidy, 1930, 1931; Scholte, 1931; Millman, 1943; Currens *et al.,* 1945). The most comprehensive study of the cardiac disease associated with the carcinoid syndrome is that of Roberts and Sjoerdsma (1964), to which the reader is recommended.

Pathology

Microscopically the essential lesion consists of focal or diffuse deposits of fibrous tissue on the luminal surface of the internal elastic lamina which are covered by apparently normal endothelium (Plate 14). The fibrous tissue is fairly cellular, numerous fibroblasts being present. There is much metachromatic ground substance which on electron microscopy has been interpreted as young collagen (Cosh *et al.,* 1959). MacDonald and Robbins (1957) have stressed the occurrence of mast cells in the lesions and there also occur some blood vessels around which are found a few lymphocytes and plasma cells. 'Spaces' containing small hyperchromatic nuclei also occur in these fibrous deposits. Elastic fibres are absent.

Distribution of the fibrous lesions and their effects

The whitish-yellow, glistening smooth deposits involve the right side of the heart more commonly than the left (Plate 15). They are frequently found on the arterial aspect of the pulmonary valve cusps, on the ventricular aspect of the posterior and septal leaflets of the tricuspid valve and on both aspects of the tricuspid anterior cusp. When the tricuspid valve is involved, then fibrous deposits are often found in the right atrium, sometimes on the internal lining of the great veins and the coronary sinus. Plaques of fibrous tissue may almost line the right ventricle, though 'white-capping' of the papillary muscles and coating of the chordae tendineae is more common. Lesions are not usually found in the pulmonary arteries or veins.

The fibrous tissue deposits tend to cause constriction of both the tricuspid and pulmonary valves, the leaflets of which become rigid and fixed. However, in the case of the pulmonary valve, stenosis is usually the predominant lesion, though some regurgitation is occasionally present. The tricuspid valve is fixed open and so regurgitation is usually predominant, though some functional stenosis of the tricuspid valve is in my experience more common than the detection of pulmonary incompetence. Maybe the predominance of stenosis or incompetence in these two valves is a reflection of the initial size of the two valve rings.

Lesions on the left side of the heart, though less common than those on the right, undoubtedly occur. Usually the lesions on the right side of the heart predominate and are accompanied by lesions on the left (Scholte, 1931; Bean *et al.,* 1955; Hand *et al.,* 1958; Bean and Funk, 1959; Thorson, 1958). However, Roberts and Sjoerdsma (1964) do not consider that in these latter cases the case for carcinoid lesions on the left side of the heart is certain. They are absolutely prepared, however, to accept the case described by McKusick (1956) in which lesion of pulmonary and tricuspid valves were associated with lesions of the mitral valve and aortic valve, but this patient had a patent foramen ovula-type atrial septal defect. A similar case was described by Fischer and Lindeneg (1958).

In terms of the aetiology of the carcinoid heart lesions it is of interest to examine its occurrence in relation to bronchial carcinoid tumours. There is described one unique case, that of Von Bernheimer and his colleagues (1960). This case had a non-metastatic bronchial carcinoid tumour with fibrous plaques on the intima of the pulmonary veins and also on the mitral and aortic valves without apparent involvement of either the tricuspid or pulmonary valves or the chambers of the right side of heart. From examination of the reports of their cases with bronchial carcinoid, Roberts and Sjoerdsma (1964) consider that three had equivocal changes on the right side of the heart and two on the left, one of whom had, in addition, an atrial septal defect.

Three of the nine cases which Roberts and Sjoerdsma themselves described had definite carcinoid fibrous lesions in the left side of the heart. In all, the mitral valve was to a greater or lesser extent involved and in one case there was a carcinoid fibrous plaque in the aorta. In these patients plaques were also found on the endocardium of the left ventricle. All three patients had small intestinal primary tumours with hepatic metastatic spread.

Clinical presentation

The precise clinical diagnosis of carcinoid heart disease is not easy. It is rare that one will be faced with functionally important and clinically apparent left-sided endocardial lesions, so that the practical problem is the diagnosis of right-sided cardiac lesions.

The most common physical signs requiring interpretation are abnormal jugular venous pulsation and precordial murmurs. Both of these signs vary from time to time, the changes probably depending upon the haemodynamic state which is so variable according to the presence or absence of flushing at the time of examination. Certainly during a flush, when the cardiac output increases, both the abnormal jugular venous pulsation and the precordial murmurs usually become more obvious and may become apparent for the first time.

The jugular venous pulse may show greatly accentuated 'v' waves indicating functionally important tricuspid incompetence or giant 'a' waves indicating tricuspid stenosis. Even in the presence of these abnormal waves the relevant tricuspid murmurs may be difficult to hear. On the other hand, a pansystolic murmur over the lower end of sternum conducted to the right and to the left of the sternum increasing in intensity during inspiration may be heard and indicates tricuspid incompetence. A tricuspid diastolic murmur, usually most obvious during flushing, may indicate tricuspid stenosis. These tricuspid murmurs are, in my experience, by no means typical of those heard in either chronic rheumatic disease of the tricuspid valve or in functional incompetence of the tricuspid valve. Perhaps this is because of the variability in cusp distortion caused by the carcinoid fibrotic lesion.

A systolic murmur over the upper part of the left sternal edge, harsh in quality and of usually rather low intensity, often indicates pulmonary stenosis. Although with pulmonary stenosis and tricuspid incompetence one would expect marked right ventricular hypertrophy, and Roberts and Sjoerdsma (1964) remark on this, right ventricular hypertrophy of a marked degree is unusual in my experience.

The development of these cardiac lesions is of great interest. So often the patient presents for the first time with the cardiac lesions fully developed. Occasionally, however, one observes the development of the cardiac disease. In one personal case observed over a period of seven years, there was on initial presentation no clinical evidence of cardiac disease. This patient had a primary ileal carcinoid with hepatic metastases, marked flushing and a little diarrhoea. Over a period of three years murmurs indicating pulmonary stenosis and tricuspid incompetence appeared, together with abnormal jugular venous pulsation. After five years a definite tricuspid diastolic murmur appeared, with clinical evidence of right ventricular enlargement, and at this stage dependent oedema requiring diuretic therapy became obvious. The degree of functional cardiac impairment is very variable. Some patients with apparently severe valvular lesions may go on for many years with little or no obvious cardiac failure, others deteriorate very quickly. I suspect that individual myocardial function is the factor determining this variability and perhaps the degree of intermittent or permanent increase in cardiac output caused by vasodilatation may also be involved.

X-ray and electrocardiographic examinations in patients with carcinoid heart disease do not reveal any specific features (Roberts and Sjoerdsma, 1964). These workers have also reviewed the haemodynamic changes in carcinoid heart disease. Right heart catheterization has revealed tricuspid insufficiency as the most common haemodynamic alteration, followed by pulmonary stenosis. Tricuspid stenosis is apparently much less common. Minimal pulmonary hypertension has been found (Charms *et al.,* 1959).

As mentioned previously, the cardiac output is frequently elevated. Such elevation may be permanent. More commonly the elevation is seen during a flushing attack (Schwaber and Lukas, 1962) and see page 54. Schneckloth *et al.* (1957) reported an elevated cardiac output in the resting state in a carcinoid patient without valvular disease. Such increases could obviously severely stress a myocardium already hampered by carcinoid valvular disease.

Pathogenesis of the cardiac lesions

Here it would be honest to state that it is not known what causes the cardiac lesions. There are certain tantalizing clues in this problem. The development of the fibrotic lesions is slow. There is not any apparent acute inflammatory endocardial lesion progressing to a chronic fibrotic lesion, as is usually the case in rheumatic heart disease. The undeniable predominance of right-sided heart lesions in cases with ileal tumours and hepatic metastases suggests that the lungs protect the left side of the heart in some way. The occasional case of a bronchial adenoma draining into the pulmonary venous circuit and producing left heart lesions, and their occurrence with atrial septal defects, also suggests a protective action of the lungs. There is the clinical impression that patients with more or less fixed cyanotic flushing are more prone to present with cardiac lesions. There is the predisposition of carcinoid patients to fibrotic lesions elsewhere as previously discussed on page 58. The distribution of the lesions and their histological features is distinctive and differs from those found in rheumatic endocarditis, congenital fibroelastosis, endomyocardial fibrosis and collagen disease (Roberts and Sjoerdsma, 1964). There is no evidence of superficial platelet disposition on the endocardium and no evidence of progression from acuteness to chronicity on microscopic examination. From patient to patient there is great uniformity of the lesions.

The intact endothelium, intact internal elastic lamina and endocardium, the deposition of the fibrotic tissue between the two layers, the occurrence of the lesions in areas of excessive blood turbulence or in the paths of regurgitant streams of blood, suggest that something in the blood, aided by superficial friction or prolonged bathing, initiates the lesions. If such a substance is responsible, it seems it must pass through the endothelium and stimulate the growth of fibrous tissue in the subendothelial layer and it probably does not pass through the internal elastic lamina.

What might such an agent be? Both 5HT (Spector and Willoughby, 1964) and bradykinin (Lewis, 1964) have been implicated as mediators of inflammatory processes, and 5HT is known to influence the activity of fibroblasts (Highton and Garrett, 1963). Yet chronic infusions of 5HT in animals have failed to reproduce the cardiac lesions (Waldenström, 1958). This is not absolute evidence against 5HT being responsible though, because of dose, species and other variables. The occurrence of endomyocardial fibrosis in an area of Uganda where the staple diet is plantain, which contains large amounts of 5HT, led McKinney and Crawford (1965) to find that it is possible to produce fibrotic lesions in the hearts of guinea pigs by giving them plantain diets. Spatz (1965) injected 5HT and a hepatotoxic agent into tryptophan deficient guinea pigs and also produced fibrotic lesions in the heart. There is no doubt, however, that the cardiac lesions produced by these manoeuvres *differ* from the cardiac lesions of the carcinoid syndrome in anatomical distribution, tissues of the heart affected and histological appearance. There are no studies directly relating increased bradykinin formation to carcinoid heart disease.

Alternative aetiological speculations include an 'autoimmune' process recurring in the endocardium and Van der Geld *et al.* (1966) have demonstrated cardiac antibodies in the presence of carcinoid heart disease. Also there is the finding, true so far only demonstrated in the brain, that certain metabolites of 5HT might be strongly bound to tissue protein and it is possible that such binding might initiate fibroblastic tissue change. If the analogy of release of catecholamines from adrenal medullary tissue is taken, then beside 5HT, various proteins akin to chromogranins and also ATP might be released and might have pharmacological effects. there are many areas yet to be explored.

Pregnancy and the carcinoid syndrome

Because of the toxic effect of 5HT on the foetus and placenta of pregnant animals (see Southgate and Sandler, 1968) it is worth noting that Reddy *et al.* (1963) have reported five pregnancies in women with the carcinoid syndrome. In all cases labour was premature, the foetus was stillborn or died after birth, and in one case multiple congenital abnormalities were present. Southgate and Sandler, 1968, report one similar case and one case in which pregnancy was uneventful.

REFERENCES

Adamson, A. R., Grahame-Smith, D. G., Peart, W. S. and Starr, M. (1969). Pharmacological blockade of carcinoid flushing provoked by catecholamines and alcohol. *Lancet*, **2**, 293.

Bates, H. R. and Clark, R. F. (1963). Observations on the pathogenesis of carcinoid heart disease and the tanning of fluorescent fibrin by 5-hydroxytryptamine and caeruloplasmia. *Am. J. Clin. Path.* **39**, 46.

Bean, W. B. and Funk, D. (1959). The vasculocardiac syndrome of the metastatic carcinoid. *Arch. Int. Med.* **103**, 189.

Bean, W. B., Olch, D. and Weinberg, H. B. (1955). The syndrome of carcinoid and acquired valve lesions of the right side of the heart. *Circulation,* **12**, 1.

Bennett, A. and Whitney, B. (1966). A pharmacology study of the human gastrointestinal tract. *Gut*, **7**, 307.

Black, W. C. and Haffner, H. E. (1968). Diffuse hyperplasia of gastric argyrophil cells and multiple carcinoid tumours. *Cancer*, **21**, 1080.

Boullin, D. J. (1964). Observations on the significance of 5-hydroxytryptamine in relation to the peristaltic reflex of the rat. *Brit. J. Pharmacol.* **23**, 14.

Bulbring, E. and Gershon, M. D. (1968). Serotonin participation in the vagal inhibitory pathway to the stomach. *Adv. Pharmacol.* **6A**, 323.

Burkes, T. F. and Long, J. P. (1966). 5-hydroxytryptamine release into dog intestinal vasculature. *Am. J. Physiol.* **211**, 619.

Carr, R. J. and Biswas, B. K. (1966). Methysergide and retroperitoneal fibrosis. *Brit. Med. J.* **2**, 1116.

Cassidy, M. A. (1930). Abdominal carcinomatosis with probable adrenal involvement. *Proc. Roy. Soc. Med.* **24**, 139.

Cassidy, M. A. (1931). Post-mortem finding in case shown on October 10, 1930 as one of abdominal carcinomatosis associated with probable adrenal involvement. *Proc. Roy. Soc. Med.* **24**, 920.

Charms, B. L., Kohn, P., Applebaum, H. I. and Geller, J. (1959). Haemodynamic studies in a case of carcinoid cardiovascular disease. *Circulation,* **20**, 208.

Cosh, J., Cates, J. E. and Pugh, D. W. (1959). Carcinoid heart disease. *Brit. Heart. J.* **21**, 369.

Currens, J. H., Kinney, T. D. and White, P. D. (1945). Pulmonary stenosis with intact interventricular septum: report of eleven cases. *Am. Heart J.* **30**, 491.

Dockerty, M. B. and Scheifley, C. H. (1955). Metastasising carcinoid. Report of an unusual case with episodic cyanosis. *Am. J. Clin. Pathol.* **25**, 770.

Eber, M. and Schauer, A. (1959). Morphological and experimental studies on fibrosis formation in carcinoid. *Beitr. Pathol. Anat. Allegm. Pathol.* **121**, 375.

Engleman, K., Lovenberg, W. and Sjoerdsma, A. (1967). Inhibition of serotonin synthesis by parachlorophenylalanine in patients with the carcinoid syndrome. *New Eng. J. Med.* **277**, 1103.

Fabricius, J., Jensen, K. and Poulsen, H. E. (1958). Metastasising carcinoid: results of cardiac catheterisation and autopsy in a case previously published. *Danish Med. Bull.* **5**, 237.

Fadell, E. J. and Denham, R. M. (1966). Carcinoid heart disease with bilateral ventricular endocardial sclerosis. *Am. J. Cardiol.* **17**, 259.

Feldberg, W. and Toh, C. C. (1953). Distribution of 5-hydroxytryptamine (Serotonin, Enteramine) in the wall of the digestive tract. *J. Physiol.* **119**, 352.

Fischer, S. and Lindeneg, O. (1958). Cardiac changes in argentaffinosis. *Acta path. et microbiol. Scandinav.* **44**, 128.

Fishlock, D. J. and Parks, A. G. The effect of 5HT on the human ileum and colon *in vitro. Brit. J. Pharmacol.* **28**, 164.

Grahame-Smith, D. G. (1968). The Carcinoid Syndrome. *Am. J. Cardiol.* **21**, 376.

Hale, J. F. and Lane-Mitchell, W. (1964). The Carcinoid Syndrome. Case report and review. *Central African J. Med.* **10**, 162.

Hallén, A. (1964). Fibrosis in the carcinoid syndrome. *Lancet,* **1**, 746.

Hand, A. M., McCormick, W. F. and Lemb, G. (1958). Malignant carcinoid tumour. A case report with discussion of systemic manifestations. *Am. J. Clin. Path.* **30**, 47.

Haverback, B. J. and Davidson, J. (1958). Serotonin and the gastrointestinal tract. *Gastroenterology,* **35**, 570.

Hedinger, C. and Gloor, R. (1954). Metastasierende Dünndarmkarzinoide, Tricuspidalklappenveränderungen und Pulmonalstenose ein neues Syndrom. *Schweiz. Med. Wochschr.* **84**, 942.

Hedinger, C., Hardmeier, T. and Funk, H. U. (1966). Das argentaffine system des Verdauungstraktes bei Carcinoidsyndrom. *Arch. Path. Anat. Physiol.* **340**, 304.

Hendrix, T. R., Atkinson, M., Clifton, J. A. and Inglefinger, F. J. (1957). The effect of 5-hydroxytryptamine on intestinal motor function in man. *Am. J. Med.* **23**, 886.

Highton, T. C. and Garrett, M. H. (1963). Some effects of serotonin and related compounds on human collagen. *Lancet,* **1**, 1234.

Hilton, S. M. and Lewis, G. P. (1956). The relationship between glandular activity, bradykinin formation and functional vasodilatation in the submandibular salivary gland. *J. Physiol.* **174**, 400.

House, H. C. and Hermann, R. E. (1965). Functioning malignant carcinoid: A review of nine cases. *Cleveland Clinic Quarterly,* **32**, 217.

Jatlow, P. and Rice, J. (1964). Bronchial adenoma with hyperserotoninaemia, biventricular valvular lesions and osteoblastic metastases. *Am. J. Clin. Path.* **42**, 285.

Kowlessar, O. D., Williams, R. C., Law, D. H. and Sleisenger, M. H. (1958). Urinary excretion of 5-hydroxyindole acetic acid in diarrhoeal states with special reference to non-tropical sprue. *New Eng. J. Med.* **259**, 340.

Kowlessar, O. D., Law, D. H. and Sleisenger, M. H. (1959). Malabsorption syndrome associated with carcinoid tumour. *Am. J. Med.* **27**, 673.

Levine, R. J. and Sjoersdma, A. (1963). Pressor amines and the carcinoid flush. *Ann. Int. Med.* **58**, 818.

Lewis, G. P. (1964). Plasma kinins and other vasoactive compounds in acute inflammation. *Ann. New York Acad. Sci.* **116**, 847.

Linell, F. and Månsson, K. (1966). On the prevalence and incidence of carcinoids in Malmo. *Acta Med. Scand.* **179** (Suppl.) 377.

MacDonald, R. A. and Robbins, S. L. (1957). Pathology of the heart in the carcinoid syndrome. A comparative study. *Arch. Path.* **63**, 103.

MacDonald, R. A. (1956). A study of 356 carcinoids of the gastrointestinal tract. Report of four new cases of the carcinoid syndrome. *Am. J. Med.* **21**, 867.

Mattingly, T. W. and Sjoerdsma, A. (1956). The cardiovascular manifestations of functioning carcinoid tumours. *Mod. Cone. Cardivasi. Dis.* **25**, 7.

McKinney, B. and Crawford, M. A. (1965). Fibrosis in guinea pig heart produced by plantain diet. *Lancet,* **2**, 880.

McKusick, V. A. (1956). Carcinoid dardiovascular disease. *Bull. Johns Hopkins Hosp.* **98**, 13.

Melmon, K. L., Sjoerdsma, A., Oates, J. A. and Laster, L. (1963). Treatment of malabsorption and diarrhoea of the carcinoid syndrome with methysergide. *Gastroenterology,* **48**, 18.

Melmon, K., Lovenberg, W. and Sjoerdsma, A. (1965). Identification of lysyl-bradykinin as the peptide formed *in vitro* by carcinoid tumour kallikrein. *Clin. Chim. Acta.* **12**, 292.

Mengel, C. E. (1965). Therapy of the malignant carcinoid syndrome. *Ann. Int. Med.* **62**, 587.

Millman, S. (1943). Tricuspid stenosis and pulmonary stenosis complicating carcinoid of the intestine with metastases to the liver. *Am. Heart J.* **25**, 391.

Misiewicz, J. J., Waller, S. L. and Eisner, M. (1966). Motor responses of the human gastrointestinal tract to 5-hydroxytryptamine *in vivo* and *in vitro*. *Gut,* **7**, 208.

Nash, D. T. and Brin, M. (1964). Malabsorption in malignant carcinoid with normal 5HIAA. *New York J. Med.* **64**, 1128.

Oates, J. A., Pettinger, W. A. and Doctor, R. B. (1966). Evidence for the release of bradykinin in the carcinoid syndrome. *J. Clin. Invest.* **45**, 173.

Oates, J. A., Melmon, K., Sjoerdsma, A., Gillespie, L. and Mason, D. T. (1964). Release of a kinin peptide in the carcinoid syndrome. *Lancet,* **1**, 514.

Oates, J. A. and Butler, T. C. (1967). Pharmacologic and endocrine aspects of the carcinoid syndrome. *Adv. Pharmacol.* **5**, 109.

Olesen, K. H. Carcinoid 1 Tyndtarmen. Tilfaelde med Livermatastaser Højresidig Hjerteklapfejl og en usaedvanlig form for cyanose—et nyt syndrom.

Page, I. H. (1968). *Serotonin.* Year Book Medical Publishers Inc., Chicago.

Page, I. H. and McCubbin, J. W. (1953). Variable arterial pressure response to serotonin in laboratory animals and man. *Circulat. Res.* **1**, 354.

Peart, W. S., Andrews, T. H. and Robertson, J. I. S. (1959). Facial flushing produced in patients with carcinoid syndrome by intravenous adrenaline and noradrenaline. *Lancet,* **2**, 715.

Reddy, D. V., Adams, F. H. and Baird, C. (1963). Teratogenic effects of serotonin. *J. Paediat.* **63**, 394.

Roberts, W. C. and Sjoerdsma, A. (1964). The cardiac disease associated with the carcinoid syndrome. (Carcinoid heart disease). *Am. J. Med.* **36**, 5.

Robertson, J. I. S., Peart, W. S. and Andrews, T. M. (1962). The mechanism of facial flushes in the carcinoid syndrome. *Quart. J. Med.* **21**, 103.

Said, S. I. and Mutt, V. (1970). Potent peripheral and splanchnic vasodilator peptide from normal gut. *Nature.* **225**, 863.

Sandler, M. (1968). 5-hydroxyindoles and the carcinoid syndrome. *Advances in Pharmacology.* **6B**.

Sandler, M., Karim, S. M. M. and Williams, E. D. (1968). Prostaglandins in amine-peptide-secreting tumours. *Lancet.* **2**, 1053.

Schneckloth, R., Page, I. H., Del Greco, F. and Corcoran, A. C. (1957). Effects of serotonin antagonists in normal subjects and patients with carcinoid tumours. *Circulation* **16**, 523.

Scholte, A. J. (1931). Ein Fall von Angioma telangiectaticum Cates mit chronischer Endokarditis und malignem Dünndarmcarcinoid. *Beitr. path. Anat.* **86**, 440.

Schwaber, J. R. and Lukas, D. S. (1962). Hyperkinaemia and cardiac failure in the carcinoid syndrome. *Am. J. Med.* **32**, 846.

Schwartz, F. D., Dunea, G. and Kark, R. M. (1966). Methysergide and retroperitoneal fibrosis. *Am. Heart. J.* **72**, 843.

Southgate, J. and Sandler, M. (1968). 5-hydroxyindole metabolism in pregnancy. *Adv. Pharmacol.* **6A**, 179.

Sokoloff, B. (1968). *Carcinoid and Serotonin.* Springer-Verlag, Berlin.

Stacey, R. S. (1957). Malignant carcinoid tumours. *Proc. Roy. Soc. Med.* **50**, 40.

Spatz, M. (1965). Pathogenetic studies of experimentally induced heart lesions and their relation to the carcinoid syndrome. *Lab. Invest.,* **13**, 288.

Spector, W. G. and Willoughby, D. A. (1964). Vasoactive amines in acute inflammation. *Am. New York Acad. Sci.* **116**, 847.

Torvik, A. (1960). Carcinoid syndrome in a primary tumour of the ovary. *Acta Pathol. Microbiol. Scand.* **48**, 81.

Thörson, A. (1958). Studies on carcinoid disease. *Acta Med. Scand.* **334**, (Suppl.) 7.

Utz, D. C., Rooke, E. D., Spittell, J. A. and Bartholomew, L. G. (1965). Retroperitoneal fibrosis in patients taking methysergide. *J. Am. Med. Assoc.* **191**, 983.

Van der Geld, Pectoom, F., Somers, K. and Kanyerezi, B. R. (1966). Immunological and serological studies in endomyocardial fibrosis. *Lancet,* **2**, 1210.

Von Bernheimer, H., Ehringer, H., Heistracher, P., Kraupp, O., Lachnit, V., Obiditsch-Mayer, I. and Wenzyl, M. (1960). Biologisch aktives, nicht metastasierendes Bronchuscarcinoid mit Linksherzsyndrom. *Wein. Klin. Wchnschr.* **72**, 867.

Waldenström, J. (1958). Clinical picture of carcinoidosis. *Gastroenterology,* **35**, 565.

Williams, E. D. and Celestin, L. R. (1962). The association of bronchial carcinoid and pluriglandular adenomatosis. *Thorax,* **17**, 120.

Zeitlin, I. J. and Smith, A. N. (1966). 5-hydroxyindoles and kinins in the carcinoid and dumping syndromes. *Lancet,* **2**, 986.

CHAPTER 6

Diagnosis

The problems encountered in diagnosis should be stated in practical terms:
1. Does the patient have the carcinoid syndrome?
2. If so, has metastatic tumour spread, particularly to the liver, occurred?
3. If metastatic spread to the liver has occurred, how deeply should one search for the primary tumour?
4. If metastatic spread to the liver has *not* occurred, where is the primary tumour?

If these questions are answered then a rational course of management can be decided upon.

The diagnosis of the carcinoid syndrome is frequently raised in patients complaining of unexplained flushing and diarrhoea and sometimes in patients with right-sided cardiac lesions and cardiac failure.

The demonstration of tumour growth, flush provocation and increased 5-hydroxyindole synthesis are the three diagnostic criteria to aim for.

The demonstration of tumour growth

Primary ileal tumours can be very difficult to demonstrate. They are frequently so small as to be impalpable and not apparent even on the most careful of barium studies. If a mass is palpable in the R.I.F. then this is likely to be due to fibrosis and matting together of bowel loops. Of course, with an ileal tumour producing the syndrome hepatic metastases are usually present. Most commonly the liver is enlarged and palpable but occasionally it is not. Radioscanning of the liver is most useful (Plate 16). Not only may it show metastatic growth in impalpable livers but shows its extent and gives information invaluable for assessing the feasibility of partial hepatectomy. If metastatic growth in the liver is present then the decision must be made on the extent of the hunt for the primary tumour. Of course it is always nice to be in command of a clinical situation and know all about the disease in the individual patient, but this may require a laparotomy to locate a primary intra-abdominal

68

tumour. Unless intestinal obstruction is a problem then a laparotomy with its risks in these patients is not justified on the grounds of curiosity alone, when liver metastases are present. In this situation I believe opening the abdomen is only justified either to relieve the local effects of tumour or in the hope that an appreciable functioning mass of tumour can be removed from the liver or elsewhere.

The position is different, however, if the carcinoid syndrome is present and confirmed, and no hepatic metastases are present. Then chest X-ray and tomography of any suspicious area, together with bronchoscopy, may be required to exclude a bronchial tumour and careful pelvic examination to exclude an ovarian tumour. Bronchial and ovarian primaries can produce the carcinoid syndrome without metastases and removal of the primary can produce a cure. If the liver by all investigations cannot be shown to contain secondaries and no extra-abdominal primary can be demonstrated, then I believe one should do a laparotomy since I have seen one case of an ileal primary producing the carcinoid syndrome associated with no gross hepatic secondaries but with large intra-abdominal lymph node metastatic growth with spread into the vertebral column. Presumably this extra-hepatic growth was draining its products into the systemic circulation and producing the syndrome. Removal of such growth may greatly relieve the symptoms.

Flush provocation

The pharmacological basis of flush provocation has already been described. If the patient has noticed flushing in response to alcohol then a measure of whisky may provoke a flush and is a useful out-patient procedure. If one wishes to be more precise, then 10 cc of ethanol in 15 cc of orange juice is usually effective in those patients who will respond to alcohol. Only about one-third of patients clearly flush in response to alcohol and the drink should be gulped and not sipped. Much more reliable is flush provocation with intravenous catecholamines, which may be successful even in patients who do not complain spontaneously of flushing. The materials required are noradrenaline or adrenaline. Solutions of these are prepared immediately prior to the test by diluting the concentrated amine to give a working solution for injection of $10 \mu g/ml$. These solutions should be thrown away after the test as they are unstable. An intravenous infusion into a forearm vein of 0.9% saline or 5% dextrose is set up to provide a potential fast flow. The lead to the I.V. needle should have a rubber sleeve close to the needle into which injections can be made.

The procedure is as follows. The drip is allowed to flow as fast as it will and a pair of forceps is clipped just proximal to the rubber sleeve. The required dose of noradrenaline or adrenaline is injected into the rubber sleeve, the forceps are removed and the infusion fluid allowed to flush the material into the circulation. After about 10 s the drip is slowed. The reaction to the I.V. catecholamine is observed and is described in detail on page 43 (see Plate 17a, b). The dosage schedule used is as follows. With noradrenaline the initial dose is 1 μg. If no flush occurs within 3 min the dose is doubled until either flushing occurs or the direct pharmacological effects of noradrenaline become obvious (i.e. hyperventilation, facial pallor, transient hypertension and reflex bradycardia). If the direct pharmacological effects are observed and no flush follows and a dose of 15-20 μg has been reached, the test is negative. The sequence with adrenaline is similar though adrenaline is usually more potent in producing a flush. The starting dose of adrenaline is again 1 μg but doses of 5-10 μg are about the maximum which can be given without unpleasant side effects. The dose of noradrenaline which produces flushing is usually between 5 and 10 μg and of adrenaline 1 to 5 μg.

I have seen this procedure fail only once to produce a flush in a patient subsequently proved to have the carcinoid syndrome. The test should be performed with care in those patients with severe carcinoid heart disease and carcinoid asthma. I would not do it in a patient with a past history of paroxysmal arrhythmia as I have seen an attack of supraventricular tachycardia induced by this procedure in a patient with the carcinoid syndrome who had had episodes of arrhythmia.

Biochemical diagnosis

The hallmark of the carcinoid syndrome is an increased urinary excretion of 5-hydroxyindoles. Although whole blood 5HT levels are frequently raised their estimation is not routinely warranted. Very rarely (and I have not seen such a case) the urinary level of 5HIAA may be normal.

Quantitative estimation of urinary 5HIAA

The ability to measure urinary 5HIAA is essential to the diagnosis of the carcinoid syndrome. The methods are described in detail in the paper by Udenfriend, Weissbach and Brodie (1958) and a modification of urinary 5HIAA estimation has been described by Macfarlane *et al.* (1956). A screening test has been described by Udenfriend and his colleagues which will pick up urinary 5HIAA excretions of over 30 mg/day. This test can be done in a matter of minutes. It is simple, avoids errors that may come about through failure of organic solvents to extract 5HIAA from the urine and is worth while doing in any suspicious case. It occasionally gives false positives and its results must always be checked by the full procedure for 5HIAA estimation.

Certain drugs and foods may interfere with urinary 5HIAA estimation. Chlorpromazine and its metabolites interfere with the development of the 5HIAA—nitrosonaphthol chromophore, and bananas, which contain 5HT, increase the excretion of 5HIAA. Patients undergoing these diagnostic tests should preferably be given no medication.

Qualitative analysis of urinary 5-hydroxyindoles

Paper chromatography of the urine and staining of the chromatogram with Ehrlich's reagent is a very useful procedure. The details have been described by Jepson (1955). In the usual case only 5HIAA and its conjugates will be visible on the chromatogram after staining. If 5HTP or 5HT as well as 5HIAA appear on the chromatogram, then an atypical tumour is present (e.g. bronchial or pancreatic). Because the urinary excretion of 5-hydroxyindoles is often very high and these compounds are subject to oxidation there are often several unidentified spots on the chromatogram. The pattern of 5-hydroxyindole excretion is usually fairly easy to discern however.

For paper chromatography to be most useful, experience in the procedure and in the chromatogram staining with Ehrlich's reagent is essential. The development of the colour of the spots is very distinctive, as is the speed of development. Standards should always be run and compared with the unknown samples.

In discussion the point is often raised as to whether in a carcinoid patient, with for instance an atypical bronchial tumour, where the main tumour product is 5HTP, the urinary 5HIAA excretion could be normal and whether, therefore, a false negative test might be present. On biochemical grounds it is extremely unlikely that an excess of 5HTP could be secreted without decarboxylation to 5HT and oxidative deamination of the 5HT with the production of 5HIAA occurring elsewhere in the body. If one feels hesitant about this conclusion then the screening test of the urine for excess production of any 5-hydroxyindole and paper chromatography of the urine will solve the problem anyway.

In summary, the diagnostic workout of the carcinoid syndrome includes the following procedures:
1. Demonstration of hepatic metastases by radioscanning.
2. Qualified search for the primary tumour.
3. Flush provocation test.
4. Examination of the urine for excess excretion of 5-hydroxyindoles by:
   (a) Screening test.
   (b) Quantitative estimation of urinary 5HIAA.
   (c) Paper chromatography of the urine.

Very few, if any, cases of the carcinoid syndrome will slip through this diagnostic net.

Estimation of blood bradykinin levels is confined to a few research laboratories and is not, as yet, a useful diagnostic procedure.

Prognosis and treatment

The eventual prognosis in the carcinoid syndrome is difficult to judge. The rate of tumour growth is important. Certainly the rate of growth of ileal primaries and their hepatic secondaries is usually slow, patients living several (5-20) years troubled by the endocrine effects of their tumour. Tumours in other sites such as the bronchus and pancreas, particularly when associated with the excretion of 5HTP and 5HT in the urine, have a much worse prognosis overall, measured in months to a year to two, and are usually associated with more vicious symptoms of the syndrome. Factors apart from the rate of tumour growth are the development of cardiac lesions and local effects of the primary tumour which also take their toll. The cardiac lesions are slowly developing but in many patients congestive cardiac failure is the eventual cause of death. The metabolic effects of severe diarrhoea, the weakening effect of recurrent flushing and the cachexia associated with the malignant disease seem to produce a complex state of affairs which also results in death. Urinary 5HIAA excretion is no guide to prognosis. Tumour growth may be rapid and fatal with excretions of less than 100 μg daily. Other patients may live for many years excreting 300-400 mg 5HIAA daily. It is not wise to make a prognosis until the patient has been observed for a year or so. I have under my care three patients whose disease dates back at least six years and who are in fair general health and who are working a full day.

Two aspects of treatment are to be considered.

First, one should consider whether it is advisable or possible to remove the primary tumour and/or secondary growth or slow tumour growth with cytotoxic drug therapy.

Secondly, the use of drugs to treat the manifestations of the syndrome forms an important part of the therapy of a condition the symptoms of which may be troublesome for many years.

Surgical treatment

If a bronchial or ovarian primary without secondaries is present then it should be removed and such removal has resulted in a cure (Waldenström, 1958). If an ileal or other gastrointestinal primary is present and accompanied by secondary growth, the removal is indicated if the primary is large or causing mechanical obstruction or if operation is being undertaken for removal of secondary growth. Even if hepatic surgery is not contemplated then abdominal exploration is sometimes worth while, since large tumour growth in abdominal lymph nodes and large ovarian metastases can occasionally be removed with symptomatic improvement (Sauer *et al.*, 1958).

But the main consideration should be given as to whether or not hepatic metastases can be removed. It is because of the usually slow growing nature of hepatic metastases that in spite of multiple and massive hepatic secondaries, partial hepatic resection is worth while. Zeegen *et al.* (1969) have reviewed this subject in some detail and the reader is referred to their paper for references. At St Mary's, Mr John Stephen has performed partial hepatic resection of the left lobe in four carcinoid patients with extremely encouraging results and from our limited experience the following points are worth making.

In patients with hepatic metastases radioscanning of the liver and coeliac angiography are important pre-operative diagnostic procedures. The multiplicity, size, distribution and blood supply of the metastases can thereby be objectively assessed. Obviously the best situation is where only one or other of the two hepatic lobes is involved by tumour. It can be difficult to be certain about this but even with tumour in both lobes it is still worth while considering partial hepatic resection if one lobe is predominantly involved. There are no rules at present to go by in selecting patients for this operation. If there seems to be a good chance of removing an amount of tumour tissue which will effectively cut down the total tumour mass by a half then it seems probable that such removal will appreciably lessen the symptoms. On the other hand, many patients are seen in whom the symptoms are not disabling and one is loath to embark on such a major procedure in these cases. If one assumes that the cardiac lesions are due to tumour secretions, however, then early tumour removal should be better than later, in an attempt to reduce carcinoid heart disease. Not all patients develop carcinoid heart disease however, and there is no way of certainly predicting which ones will do so, so that even this line of action is open to argument. At the present time I would confine hepatic resection to those patients who have apparently slowly growing hepatic secondaries and who are disabled by flushing or diarrhoea in whom the tumour mass is mainly, but not necessarily exclusively, limited to one hepatic lobe and who are not in a state of gross cachexia and ill health from the disease. I would also consider patients with carcinoid heart disease who fall into the above category, especially those troubled by dependent oedema since functionally and perhaps even structurally (Chatterjee and Heather, 1968) the cardiac state may be greatly improved by removal of tumour tissue.

Removal of hepatic metastases is also advocated in those patients whose abdominal pain can be ascribed to necrosing secondaries in the liver. This is not uncommon and surgery brings real relief.

Surgically either the right or left lobes of the liver may be removed and sometimes it is possible to shell out a large secondary deposit from the lobe which is left. Carcinoid metastases are not commonly very infiltrative and a plane of cleavage can often be found around a tumour deposit. It may at first sight appear foolhardy to remove a lobe from a liver involved with metastatic growth but liver function is remarkably well maintained in carcinoid livers despite extensive involvement with tumour. Theoretically too, there is the ability of the liver in animals, and perhaps also in man, to regenerate. Careful pre-operative preparation and post-operative care are essential. Anaesthetic problems must also be considered (see Zeegen *et al.,* 1969 for references).

An illustrative case is the following. A man aged 60 with the carcinoid syndrome due to an ileal primary which was removed in 1964, when hepatic metastases were noted, continued to have severe flushing, mild diarrhoea and developed tricuspid valvular disease. He also complained of intermittent epigastric pain, thought to be due to a necrotic metastasis in the left lobe of his enlarged liver. Episodes of paroxysmal supraventricular tachycardia associated with flushing attacks also became noticeable and his degree of disability become profound.

Radioscanning of the liver revealed an almost total absence of uptake of radioactivity by the left lobe of the liver, and coeliac angiography a displacement of the left gastric vessels around a mass in the liver.

At operation a large secondary with another smaller one was found in the left lobe of the liver which was almost totally involved by tumour. The left lobe of the liver was removed. During the post-operative course the patient had severe jaundice of a combined hepatocellular-cholestatic type and a short episode of hepatic encephalopathy. He made a complete recovery however and is now free of flushing and diarrhoea. The cardiac lesions one year later are virtually unchanged but he has had no further episodes of arrhythmia. Flush provocation tests are now negative and his urinary 5HIAA excretion has fallen to normal levels from pre-operative levels of 154 mg/day.

In three other cases treated by removal of the left lobe of the liver, there have been no complications post-operatively of liver failure and although complete removal of hepatic metastases in these latter patients has not been possible, their symptoms have been greatly improved and in two the urinary 5HIAA excretions lowered respectively from 300 to 29 mg/day and 500 to 100 mg/day; in the third, despite symptomatic improvement, the urinary 5HIAA excretion has remained unchanged. There is no doubt that such operations offer the greatest relief for patients and that an aggressive surgical policy is indicated.

Cytotoxic drug therapy

Mengel (1965) has reviewed his experience in treating the malignant carcinoid syndrome with cyclophosphamide and 5-fluorouracil. Undoubtedly these drugs have a cytotoxic effect upon the tumour cells as shown by a lessening of hepatic enlargement and a change in the excretion pattern of 5-hydroxyindoles in the urine, suggesting tumour necrosis. Subsequent to treatment the 5HIAA urinary excretion was diminished. Unfortunately in the cases he reported there appears to have been little worthwhile clinical improvement. This has also been my experience with oral cyclophosphamide and intravenous vinblastine. This latter drug was given to one patient because the molecular structure of this drug contains an indole moiety and it was hoped that it might be selectively concentrated by the tumour which appears to be avid for tryptophan.

There are also some reports of the effects of infusing cytotoxic drugs into the hepatic artery. Murray-Lyon *et al.* (1970) have reported three patients with mid-gut carcinoids treated by regional infusion of the liver with 5-fluorouracil. They suggest the following regimen. First infusion of 5-fluorouracil into the hepatic artery to decrease the function of the hepatic metastases prior to ligation of the hepatic artery. Ligation of the hepatic artery causes tumour necrosis but in one of their cases produced a massive release of vasoactive materials from the tumour with severe symptoms and it is for this reason they advise prior treatment with 5-fluorouracil before hepatic artery ligation. After ligation of the hepatic artery infusion of 5-fluorouracil into a tributary of the portal vein is carried out to treat any areas of surviving tumour tissue. In two of their patients remissions of the carcinoid syndrome were achieved for five months with recurrence of minor symptoms at 12 and 16 months.

With the agents at present available it seems unlikely that the large metastases usually present in the liver will be amenable to complete destruction, by either oral or regional cytotoxic drug therapy.

Pharmacological therapy

There have been a bewildering number of drugs used in the therapy of the carcinoid syndrome but only a few are worth while considering. This is best done in relationship to the theoretical scheme presented in Fig. 12, which shows the synthesis, release and action of the known pharmacologically active substances produced by the tumour and sites of potential therapeutic attack.

Inhibition of synthesis

5HT

α-methyldopa (MD) was the first drug used in an attempt to inhibit the synthesis of 5HT by blocking the conversion of 5HTP to 5HT. Unfortunately, although it does this *in vivo* (Oates and Sjoerdsma, 1962)

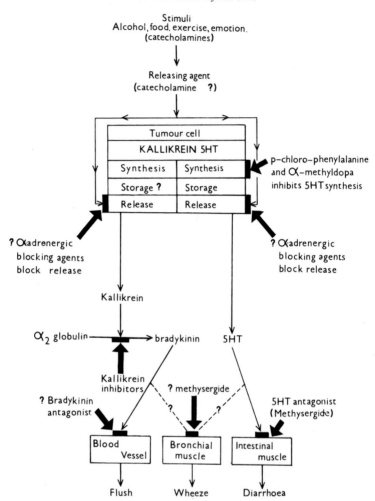

Fig. 12. Scheme of the pharmacology of the carcinoid syndrome. Central to this scheme is the tumour cell synthesizing kallikrein and 5HT (serotonin). The tumour stores and releases these substances with presumably production of the main symptoms as shown towards the bottom of the scheme. Stimuli, probably through the mediation of a catecholamine, cause release of materials from the tumour and the action of these catecholamines may be blocked by alpha-adrenergic blocking agents. On the other hand one can inhibit synthesis of 5HT most effectively with para-chlorophenylalanine and less effectively with alpha-methyldopa. Kallikrein inhibitors so far have not been useful in preventing the production of bradykinin in this syndrome. Methysergide is the most effective treatment of the diarrhoea in the carcinoid syndrome and must at present be presumed to act by antagonizing 5HT. No effective bradykinin antagonist is yet known. It may be that methysergide blocks the action of 5HT to produce broncho-constriction. The thick black arrows leading to black blocks indicate theoretical sites of attack with various forms of therapy.

its effect is partial. It seems unlikely on the evidence available that its occasional effect in relieving flushing is due to its action to inhibit the synthesis of 5HT which is probably involved only to a minor extent in the production of the flush, for improvement has been noted in patients excreting mainly 5HIAA at doses not producing an obvious increase in urinary 5HTP. It is possible that MD acts by interfering with the action of catecholamines to release flush-producing substances from the tumour cells.

The use of MD is suggested in those patients with a cyanotic type of flush, particularly if accompanied by hyperventilation. In these patients doses of 2G a day may be effective.

Parachlorophenylalanine (PCP)

The effect of PCP to inhibit the 5-hydroxylation of tryptophan was described by Koe and Weissman (1966). Engleman *et al.* (1967) showed that this compound was an effective inhibitor of 5HT synthesis in the carcinoid syndrome. Although, as expected, it has little effect upon the flushing, it does relieve the diarrhoea. More striking, however, is its occasional dramatic effect to improve the patient's appetite, vigour and well being (Grahame-Smith. Unpublished observations). The drug is used in doses of up to 4 G/day but at the time of writing it is not generally available. In Fig. 13 is shown its effect to decrease the urinary excretion of 5HIAA in 3 patients with the carcinoid syndrome.

Kallikrein and bradykinin

Although Trasylol, a commercial kallikrein inhibitor, will inhibit carcinoid tumour kallikrein *in vitro* (Melmon *et al.,* 1965), infusion of large amounts of Trasylol failed to prevent flushing induced by catecholamines and spontaneous flushing in a patient with carcinoid syndrome (Grahame-Smith *et al.,* 1964). The failure of this investigative therapy is at present unexplained and speculation is unwarranted.

Prevention of release of active substances from the tumour

Phenoxybenzamine

On pages 58-60 are described the investigations which suggest that catecholamines, certain foods, excitement, exercise and alcohol all provoke flushing by their action in releasing kallikrein and possibly 5HT from tumour cells. The effects of catecholamines and alcohol may sometimes be inhibited by the administration of phenoxybenzamine 10-20 mg t.d.s., and a quite definite diminution in the number and

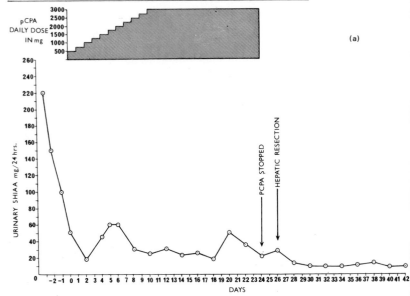

Mr. A.M.CARCINOID. EFFECT OF PCPA AND HEPATIC RESECTION ON URINARY 5HIAA

(a)

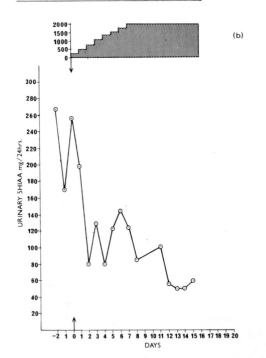

Mr. G.S.CARCINOID EFFECT PCPA ON URINARY 5HIAA

(b)

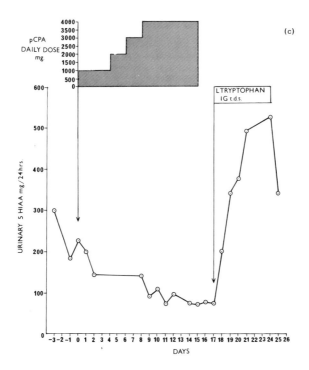

Fig. 13. The effect of para-chlorophenylalanine on urinary 5HIAA excretion in patients with metastasising ileal argentaffinomas.

(a) Male patient with the carcinoid syndrome. Excretion of 5HIAA variable between 100 and 240 mg per 24 h. The response to para-chlorophenylalanine was remarkably swift and by the time a dosage of 2.5 G daily had been reached the excretion of 5HIAA was reduced to about 20 mg per 24 h. On day 24 of para-chlorophenylalanine administration the drug was stopped and two days later he had a resection of the left lobe of the liver. Thereafter his 5HIAA excretion was about 10 mg per 24 h, i.e. within normal limits.

(b) A male patient with the carcinoid syndrome. Again the response to para-chlorophenylalanine was rapid and on 2 G per day of the substance 5HIAA excretion had fallen from between 160 and 270 mg per day to about 50 to 60 mg per day.

(c) A woman with the carcinoid syndrome. Para-chlorophenylalanine reduced the 5HIAA excretion from its high value of 150 to 300 mg per 24 h to constantly lower values of 75 mg per 24 h at a dosage of 4 G daily. Enzyme inhibition in this patient was reversible as shown by the effect of L-tryptophan to cause a gross increase in the excretion of 5HIAA starting two days after stopping the para-chlorophenylalanine. Undoubtedly the tumour is dependent upon a supply of L-tryptophan for its function in producing serotonin.

severity of flushing attacks can sometimes be achieved with this α-adrenergic blocking agent. Its side effects, such as dizziness and nasal obstruction, limit its use. Patients not infrequently become refractory to its effect. Propranolol appears to be equivocally effective in diminishing flushing (Ludwig *et al.*, 1968) and so far I have not observed a useful effect.

Inhibition of action of active substances released from the tumour

Methysergide

This drug, which is a potent antagonist of 5HT, is frequently effective in treating the diarrhoea of the carcinoid syndrome (Peart and Robertson, 1961), and is the drug of first choice in treating severe carcinoid diarrhoea. Its effect is obvious within one day. Doses employed vary between 3-8 mg daily given in three divided doses. Little or no effect upon flushing is noted. The side effects of this drug, noted in relation to its use in the treatment of migraine (Graham, 1964) include vascular spasm and retroperitoneal fibrosis. The risk of these toxic effects must be weighed against its potential benefit.

Other 5HT antagonists such as cyproheptadine and a new 5HT antagonist, BC 105 (a benzocycloheptathiophene derivative) (Loong *et al.*, 1968) may also be effective in controlling diarrhoea and occasionally and unexpectedly flushing.

Other agents

The flushing caused by bronchial tumours is often very severe and distressing and in these cases prednisone in doses of about 20 mg daily can bring about dramatic relief. In some cases it is possible to titrate the dose against its effect. The mechanism of action is unknown but when successful not only does it relieve the flushing in bronchial carcinoids but also the hyperdynamic cardiac state, the facial swelling, associated diarrhoea and general distress. Whether it prevents the release of active substances from the tumour or blocks their action is for future investigation to sort out. It is odd that it is singularly ineffective in preventing flushing or diarrhoea caused by the more common gastrointestinal carcinoids.

Chlorpromazine, which has a multiplicity of pharmacological actions, may occasionally control flushing. Codeine phosphate may be used in mild diarrhoea. Nicotinic acid should be used for the treatment of the pellegra-like skin lesions. Various other forms of therapy which have not yet been fully assessed have been reviewed by Sokoloff (1968).

Heart failure should be treated by conventional therapy. Oedema may respond dramatically to spironolactone. Wheezing, if very troublesome, is best treated with an isoprenaline or salbutamol aerosol, and this treatment does not provoke flushing.

REFERENCES

Chatterjee, K. and Heather, J. G. (1968). Carcinoid heart disease from primary ovarian tumours. *Am. J. Med.* **45**, 643.

Engleman, K., Lovenberg, W. and Sjoerdsma, A. (1967). Inhibition of serotonin synthesis by parachlorophenylalanine in patients with the carcinoid syndrome. *New. Eng. J. Med.* **277**, 1103.

Graham, J. R. (1964). Methysergide for the prevention of headache. Experience in five hundred patients over three years. *New Engl. J. Med.* **270**, 67.

Grahame-Smith, D. G., Peart, W. S. and Ferriman, D. G. (1965). Carcinoid Syndrome. *Proc. Roy. Soc. Med.* **58**, 701.

Jepson, J. B. (1955). Paper chromatography of urinary indoles. *Lancet,* **2**, 1009.

Koe, B. K. and Weissman, A. (1966). p-Chlorophenylalanine. A specific depletor of brain serotonin. *J. Pharmacol. & Exper. Therap.* **154**, 499.

Loong, S. C., Lance, J. W., Rawle, K. C. T. (1968). The control of flushing and diarrhoea in carcinoid syndrome by an antiserotonin agent, BC 105. *Med. J. Aust.* **55**, 845.

Ludwig, G. D., Cushard, W., Bartuska, D., Franco, R. and Chaykin, L. (1968). Effects of beta-adrenergic blockade in the carcinoid syndrome (abstr.). *Ann. Int. Med.* **68**, 1188.

Macfarlane, P. S., Dalgliesh, C. C., Dutton, R. W., Lennox, B., Nyhus, L. M. and Smith, A. N. (1956). Endocrine aspects of argentaffinoma. *Scot. Med. J.* **1**, 148.

Melmon, K., Lovenberg, W. and Sjoerdsma, A. (1965). Identification of lysyl-bradykinin as the peptide formed *in vitro* by carcinoid tumour kallikrein. *Clin. Chim. Acta.* **12**, 292.

Mengel, C. E. (1965). Therapy of the malignant carcinoid syndrome. *Ann. Int. Med.* **62**, 587.

Murray-Lyon, I. M., Dawson, J. L., Parsons, V. A., Rake, M. O., Blendis, L. M., Laws, J. W. and Williams, R. (1970). Treatment of secondary hepatic tumours by ligation of hepatic artery and infusion of cytotoxic drugs. *Lancet,* **2**, 172.

Oates, J. A. and Sjoerdsma, A. (1962). A unique syndrome associated with secretion of 5-hydroxytryptophan by metastatic gastric carcinoids. *Am. J. Med.* **32**, 333.

Peart, W. S. and Robertson, J. I. S. (1961). The effect of a serotonin antagonist (UML 491) in carcinoid disease. *Lancet,* **2**, 1172.

Reddy, D. V., Adams, F. H., Baird, C. (1963). Teratogenic effects of serotonin. *J. Pediat.* **63**, 394.

Sauer, W. G., Dearing, W. H. and Flock, E. V. (1958). Diagnosis and clinical management of functioning carcinoids. *J. Amer. Med. Ass.* **168**, 139.

Sokoloff, B. (1968). *Carcinoid and Serotonin.* Springer-Verlag, Berlin.

Southgate, J. and Sandler, M. (1968). 5-hydroxyindole metabolism in pregnancy. *Adv. Pharmacol.* **6B**, 179.

Udenfriend, S., Weissbach, H. and Brodie, B. B. (1958). Assay of serotonin and related metabolites, enzymes and rugs. *Methods, Biochem. Anal.* 6, 95.

Waldenström, J. (1958). Clinical picture of carcinoidosis. *Gastroenterology*, 35, 565.

Zeegen, R., Rothwell-Jackson, R. and Sandler, M. (1969). Massive hepatic resection for the carcinoid syndrome. *Gut,* 10, 617.

CHAPTER 7

The Carcinoid Syndrome and Ectopic Hormone Production

Ectopic hormone production means the production of a hormone by a tissue not normally envisaged as being concerned with the production of the hormone in question. The first ectopic humoral syndrome described was that by Brown in 1928, and concerned a patient with diabetes, hirsutism, hypertension, adrenal hyperplasia and an oat cell carcinoma of the lung. This was probably a case of ectopic ACTH production. Many cases of the ectopic production of ACTH have since been described and this subject, as well as the ectopic production of other hormones, has been recently reviewed by Liddle *et al.* (1969) and by Weichert (1970) to which articles the reader is referred for references.

Suffice it here to say that ectopic ACTH production is most commonly found in association with carcinomas of the bronchus but that carcinomas of the pancreas (including islet cell tumours and carcinoid tumours), carcinomas of the thyroid, liver, prostate, ovary, breast, parotid, oesophagus, and of mediastinal tissue have also been responsible. In addition, thymomas, phaeochromocytoma, para-ganglioma, ganglioma, and benign bronchial adenoma (including carcinoid) have been implicated. Ectopic ACTH production is also associated with ectopic MSH production (β MSH). The studies reported by Liddle *et al.* (1969) suggest that biologically active ACTH produced by these tumours is structurally identical to pituitary ACTH but that the tumours also produce substances similar to the C-terminal fragment of ACTH. So far the ectopic MSH seems to be similar to pituitary MSH.

Ectopic parathyroid hormone production is also reported in various tumour types. Immunoreactive parathormone has been found in carcinomas of the lung, kidney, pancreas, colon, adrenal and parotid. The evidence that ectopic parathyroid hormone is the same as normal parathyroid hormone is based upon immunological studies.

Ectopic gonadotrophin production (i.e. gonadotrophin production not associated with either pituitary or trophoblastic tumours) has been described with hepatic carcinoma and various types of carcinomas of the lung. The clinical presentation of such cases is of either isosexual precocious puberty in the child and/or gynaecomastia in the adult male.

The production of ectopic ADH has also been frequently reported in association with anaplastic oat cell carcinomas of the bronchus but its association with a duodenal carcinoma and with pancreatic carcinomas has also been noted. Various lines of evidence suggest that ectopic ADH is similar to, if not identical with, human pituitary ADH (arginine vasopressin).

Whether or not gastrin production by non-insulin producing adenomas of the islets of Langerhans with the resulting Zollinger-Ellison syndrome should be regarded as true ectopic hormone production is a matter of debate. We cannot tell whether gastrin is produced by a rare type of islet cell normally and that this cell is then the cell of origin of the neoplasm secreting gastrin and producing the Zollinger-Ellison syndrome. Nevertheless, Gregory and his colleagues (1967) have conclusively shown that the gastrin peptides produced by these tumours have the same amino acid composition as normal human gastric gastrin.

The ectopic production of erythropoietin by cerebellar haemangioblastomas, hepatomas and phaeochromocytomas has been reported. Renal neoplasms also occasionally produce erythropoietin though this cannot be considered ectopic hormone production since the normal kidney produces erythropoietin. Studies which have been done on ectopic erythropoietin suggest that this is very similar to normal renal erythropoietin.

The position as regards ectopic TSH production is more difficult. At least fourteen patients have been reported to have hyperthyroidism in association with trophoblastic tumours. However, there are reports of a TSH-like material in normal placentas so it cannot be said whether tumours of this tissue really produce an ectopic hormone.

Equally difficult is the production of ectopic insulin by non-pancreatic neoplasms. Large retroperitoneal fibrosarcomas are sometimes associated with hypoglycaemia but it appears that only rarely can it be demonstrated that such tumours are producing ectopic insulin. We shall return to this subject later.

Whether or not the production of an ectopic hormone leads to the physical changes normally associated with excessive production of that hormone presumably depends upon how much hormone is produced and over how long. To be certain that a tumour is really producing an ectopic hormone can be difficult. It is necessary to demonstrate that excessive circulating levels of the hormone are present and usually these are not under normal feed-back inhibitory control mechanisms. A difference between the levels of the hormone in the blood entering and leaving the tumour shows that the tumour is secreting the hormone. Analysis of the tumour hormone concentrations shows whether or not the tumour is storing the hormone. Pathological and biochemical examinations of the tissue normally producing the hormone sometimes suggest that in the presence of the ectopic hormone syndrome the function of the normal gland is suppressed.

Some of these criteria have been fulfilled in regard to the ectopic hormone production by carcinoid tumours but in many cases the data is only suggestive. Nevertheless, carcinoids of fore-gut derivation have been implicated in the production of Cushing's syndrome (ectopic ACTH), Escovitz and Reingold (1961); Harrison *et al.* (1957); Sagle *et al.* (1965), and in two cases (see Liddle *et al.*, 1969) removal of a bronchial carcinoid has led to a remission of the ectopic ACTH syndrome. ACTH has also been demonstrated in a bronchial carcinoid tumour (Strott *et al.*, 1968). It is not certain whether the hyperpigmentation occasionally seen is due to excess MSH production (Fernex, 1964; Granlich and Weithoff, 1960; Melmon *et al.*, 1965; Sagle *et al.*, 1965; Sandler *et al.*, 1961). As far as I am aware, no definite evidence of the production of parathyroid hormone, ADH or gonadotrophins by a carcinoid tumour has been reported.

There is another aspect to this problem which is whether 5HT and kallikrein production by bronchial tumours producing the carcinoid syndrome is an example of ectopic hormone production. It now seems most unlikely. Several cases of oat cell carcinomas of the bronchus producing the carcinoid syndrome have been described (Azzopardi and Bellan, 1965; Kinloch *et al.*, 1965; Gowenlock *et al.*, 1964; Harrison *et al.*, 1957; Parish *et al.*, 1964; Williams and Azzopardi, 1960). In addition, Gowenlock *et al.* (1963) have detected 5HT in varying concentrations in tumour tissue from patients in whom the syndrome was absent. These matters have recently been unified. Bensch and his colleagues (1968) on the basis of electron microscopic studies have concluded that in the normal bronchus are cells resembling the intestinal Kultschitzky cell and that this cell composes both bronchial carcinoid tumours and the oat cell carcinomas, in fact they go so far as to suggest that the bronchial carcinoid is the more benign form of the oat cell carcinoma.

Insulin production by carcinoid tumours is rare but has been reported. A case reported by my colleagues and myself is presented.

Case Report

At the age of 46, this female patient had 'a growth the size of a walnut' removed from the small intestine. No further details are available. Ten years later she began to notice occasional facial flushing and increased growth of hair on the face, arms and legs, and later occasional mild diarrhoea. Soon the first attack of hypoglycaemia coma occurred and these attacks became frequent. She was admitted to the Royal Berkshire Hospital where hypoglycaemia was confirmed during one of the attacks. A laparotomy was performed. No pancreatic tumour was found but the liver was involved by multiple metastatic nodules. A biopsy of one of these showed a carcinoid tumour and she was transferred to St Mary's Hospital.

Examination revealed a thin woman who had infrequent mild erythematous flushes involving the face, neck and upper chest, occurring usually after meals. Excessive hair was present on the face, arms and legs. A large left supraclavicular lymph node was present. The B.P. was 130/80; there was no increase in jugular venous pressure. A soft pansystolic murmur was present at the lower end of the left sternal edge. The liver was enlarged 2 in below the right costal margin.

Investigations

Flushing was provoked by the intravenous administration of adrenaline 2 μg and noradrenaline 10 μg. Oral ethanol did not provoke flushing. The concentration of bradykinin in the arterial blood did not rise during flushing induced by adrenaline (non-flushing bradykinin concentrations were 2.2 ng and 2.9 ng/ml and during a flush 2.5 ng and 3.5 ng/ml). Intravenous bradykinin, 60 μg, caused the expected flush. Urinary 5-hydroxyindole acetic acid (5HIAA) excretion was 270 mg/24 h. Two dimensional paper chromatography of the urine revealed an increase in 5HIAA only. No 5-hydroxytryptamine (5HT) or 5-hydroxytryptophan (5HTP) spots were present.

The effects of a prolonged fast upon the plasma glucose and plasma immunoreactive insulin are shown in Fig. 14. After 28 h of fasting a hypoglycaemic attack occurred (plasma glucose 16 mg/100 ml). This was effectively reversed with intravenous glucose.

Thirty minutes after oral leucine (150 mg/Kg body wt) there was a rise in plasma immunoreactive insulin from 45 μU/ml to a peak level of 85 μU/ml. There was no impressive increase in plasma immunoreactive insulin in response to I.V. tolbutamide and I.V. glucagon. Glucose administration orally and I.V. did not predictably cause an increase in plasma immunoreactive insulin. The rate constants for glucose disappearance after two separate I.V. glucose tolerance tests were normal (i.e. K = 1.44 and 2.04). Low plasma glucose levels (25 mg/100 ml) were frequently associated with inappropriately high plasma immunoreactive insulin concentrations. There was no rise in plasma immunoreactive insulin concentrations during flushing provoked by I.V. adrenaline.

Other investigations aimed at discovering any ectopic hormone production—fasting plasma growth hormone concentration was 2 ng/ml; plasma cortisol after dexamethasone suppression, 4 μg/100 ml; urinary 17-hydroxycorticosteroids 5.8 mg/24 h, 17-oxosteroids 4.8 mg/24 h; plasma osmolality 285 milliosmols/litre, urinary osmolality 702 milliosmols/litre; I^{131} thyroid uptake normal, P.B.I. 6.4 μg/100 ml; serum calcium 10.2 mg/100 ml; serum inorganic phosphorus

3.1 mg/100 ml; serum alkaline phosphatase 12.0 U/100ml. Thus no gross evidence was found for excessive production of growth hormone, ACTH, TSH, ADH or parathormone. There was no overall increase in the urinary excretion of adrenal androgens. The hirsutism was not investigated further.

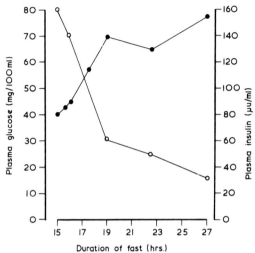

Fig. 14. Blood glucose values and the plasma level of immuno-reactive insulin in a patient with an ileal argentaffinoma producing hypoglycaemia. Fifteen hours of fasting produced a sustained fall in plasma glucose levels down to 15 mg/100 ml at which time a hypoglycaemic attack occurred. During this fall of blood glucose there was no fall in plasma insulin levels, in fact there was a paradoxical rise.

Course

The hypoglycaemic attacks became more frequent and more difficult to control by either diet or oral glucose supplements. Plasma glucose levels of 10 mg/100 ml were frequently recorded during attacks. Treatment with diazoxide was begun and the dose gradually increased to 500 mg daily in divided doses, together with frusemide 40 mg daily and bendrofluazide 10 mg daily. Fluid retention, nausea and tachycardia were very troublesome on this dose of diazoxide and it had little effect on the frequency of hypoglycaemic attacks. Prednisone 5 mg t.d.s. added to this therapy had no effect and in one of the hypoglycaemic attacks cardiac arrest occurred.

Post-mortem examination

Near the ileo-caecal valve there was a mass consisting of coiled and adherent loops of small intestine. Although the mucosa and wall of the gastrointestinal tract showed no macroscopic tumour, microscopy showed infiltration of this mass by nests and cords of carcinoid cells. These appearances are very likely due to a secondary fibrotic reaction and tumour infiltration at the site of removal of the primary tumour, which we assume was carried out in 1957. The liver was enlarged, containing multiple yellowish tumour nodules with harmorrhagic areas. Both ovaries were greatly enlarged (R 495 G and L 135 G) and appeared completely replaced by tumour. Tumour seedlings were present on the peritoneum.

The pancreas was macroscopically normal. Microscopically the number of islets was within normal limits and the islets appeared normal. Staining with the Gomori-aldehyde-fuchsin method did not show β-cell granules.

In the chest there were some enlarged tracheo-bronchial lymph nodes containing carcinoid tumour and tumour was present beneath the pleura of both lungs on microscopic examination. There was no evidence of carcinoid heart disease.

The argentaffin reaction on post-mortem material revealed scanty positive granules. The diazonium reaction on the liver biopsy at operation was markedly positive (Fig. 18).

The tumour contained 138 μg 5HT/G tissue and paper chromatography of an extract showed that 5HT was the major 5-hydroxyindole present. No 5HTP or 5HIAA was detected in the tumour. Acid ethanol extracts of the liver tissue not involved by tumour and of hepatic metastases were assayed for immunoreactive insulin. The normal liver contained 4.5 μU/G, the tumour tissue 14.5 μU/G.

From the post-mortem and histological evidence it seems safe to assume that the primary tumour in this case was an ileal argentaffinoma which was incompletely removed in 1957. The presence of an excess of 5HIAA in the urine, the absence of major amounts of 5HTP and 5HT from the urine, the absence of 5HTP in the tumour and the presence in the tumour of large amounts of 5HT are also typical of an ileal carcinoid tumour. Although at post-mortem, perhaps because of autolysis, the argentaffin stain showed only scanty positive granyles the diazonium stain on the biopsy specimen at operation showed many positively staining cells. In all these respects this was a typical ileal argentaffinoma. Flushing in this case was not accompanied by a rise in arterial plasma bradykinin levels.

The unusual feature of this case was the hypoglycaemia due to increased levels of circulating immunoreactive insulin. The question of the source of this insulin cannot be answered with absolute certainty. Although the metastatic tumour tissue contained more insulin than the normal contiguous liver the tumour concentration of insulin was low compared with the insulin concentrations found in normal pancreas and

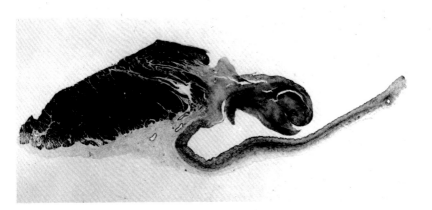

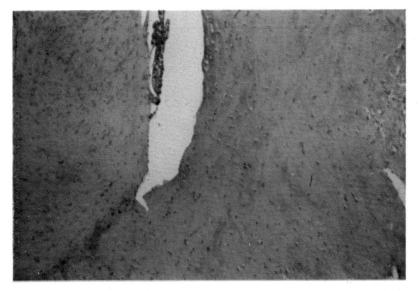

Plate 14. Histology of the tricuspid valve post mortem in a patient with carcinoid heart disease.

(a) Note the superficial deposition of fibrous tissue on the distal aspect of the valve cusp and

(b) under high power magnification its homogeneous appearance.

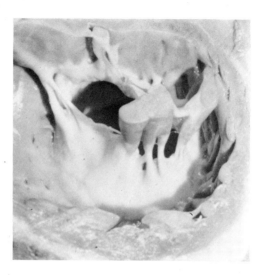

Plate 15. Macroscopic appearance of valves affected by carcinoid heart disease. This shows the tricuspid valve of a patient with a metastatic ileal argentaffinoma. Note the gross superficial fibrosis capping the capillary muscles and involving the under surface of the valve causing its distortion and incompetence.

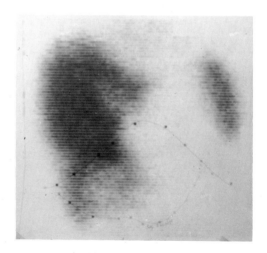

Plate 16. Liver scan of a patient with a metastatic bronchial carcinoid. Note the multiple filling defects in the enlarged right lobe of the liver and the lack of radioactivity where the left lobe of the liver should be (scan after I.V. injection of 1.3 mCi technecium 99 colloid).

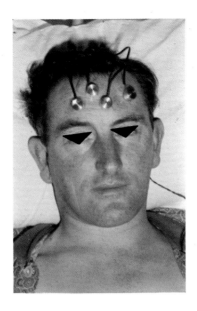

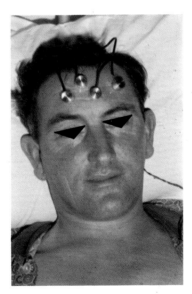

Plate 17. (a) A patient with erythematous flushing produced by metastasising ileal argentaffinoma. The brass discs on the forehead were to record skin temperature. At rest little abnormal is seen.

(b) After the injection of 10 micrograms of noradrenaline intravenously, the patient shows an erythematous flush of the face, neck and upper part of the chest.

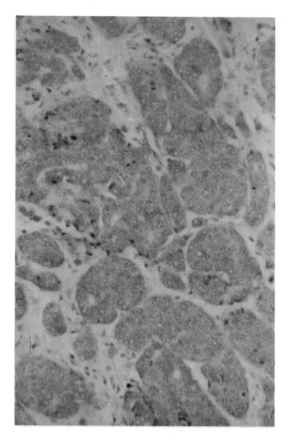

Plate 18. Diazo-stain of heptatic biopsy specimen taken from patient with ileal argentaffinoma producing hypoglycaemia. Note clumps of carcinoid cells and the presence of many positive diazo-staining cells.

insulinomas. This does not exclude the tumour as the source of insulin for it may have synthesized and quickly secreted insulin without storing it. The studies done on the control of plasma insulin levels in this patient showed that insulin levels were not decreased in response to a low plasma glucose concentration and although leucine caused a release of insulin, tolbutamide, glucagon, oral and I.V. glucose did not convincingly demonstrate insulin release. Certainly the secretion of insulin, from whatever source, was not responsive to normal controlling mechanisms. The problem which cannot be resolved on the data obtained is whether this argentaffinoma was producing the insulin or whether it was producing a substance which was stimulating the pancreas to produce insulin. It seems very likely that the tumour was producing insulin because of the associations which have been occasionally reported between carcinoid tumours, islet-cell tumours, the carcinoid syndrome, hypoglycaemia with hyperinsulinism and excess 5-hydroxyindole metabolism. In Table 10 are set out the relevant features of these cases with which the present case is compared. Examination of this Table provides a tantalizing glimpse of an association between islet cells and enterochromaffin cells and their derivatives, which can be viewed either in terms of their functional differentiation from a common embryonic parent cell and a partial return to common function on malignant change or in the context of the odd association between a β-cell adenoma and some small ileal carcinoid tumours (Table 10, case described by Schmid *et al.,* 1963). Also relevant are those tumours apparently arising from exocrine pancreatic tissue which cause the carcinoid syndrome (Peart *et al.,* 1963). There does appear to be a considerable range of tumour types involved. This probably reflects either a confusing similarity which may have an embryonic basis between islet cells and enterochromaffin cells. The tumour under discussion was very unusual in having such clear morphology and histochemical reactions and yet producing insulin.

What conclusions can be drawn from considerations of the involvement of malignant enterochromaffin cells in ectopic hormone production?

All the evidence so far shows that ectopic hormones are similar if not identical to the natural hormones. It seems probable, therefore, that normal processes are being used for the production of these hormones and that this production is *not* due to haphazard, uncontrolled, random polypeptide and enzyme protein synthesis and that by chance some of these polypeptides and enzymes have the properties of hormones or the capacity to synthesize amines. If this is so, we are observing some kind of a derepression of cellular functions which during the process of differentiation of the normal enterochromaffin cell had become repressed. It is now an axiom that cells, however specialized they have become, still contain the genetic information present in the original stem

TABLE 10

Details of cases relating carcinoid tumours, the carcinoid syndrome and insulin production

Authors	Tumour type	Argent-affinity	Carcinoid syndrome	Hypo-glycaemia	Hyper-insulinism	Tumour insulin	Pancreatic insulin	Tumour 5-hydroxyindoles	Urinary 5-hydroxyindoles
Schmid et al., 1963 (17)	Pancreatic islet cell adenoma + multiple ileal carcinoids	∓	−	+	+	N.T.	N.T.	N.T.	Normal
Gloor et al., 1964 (18)	Pancreatic islet cell	±	Diarrhoea	−	N.T.	+	+	5HT+	N.T.
Sluys et al., 1964 (19)	Pleomorphic pancreatic?-islet cell	−	+	+	N.T.	−	N.T.	−	+
Shames et al., 1968 (20)	Bronchial carcinoid	−	+	+	+	+	+	N.T.	N.T.
Appleyard & Losowsky 1970 (21)	Pancreatic adenocarcinoma (? type)	−	+	+	+	N.T.	N.T.	N.T.	5HT+ 5HIAA+
Present case	Malignant ileal argentaffinoma	+	+	+	+	+	N.T.	5HT+	5HIAA+

N.T. = Not tested.

cell from which they sprang. The most direct evidence for this is the work of Gurdon and Uehlinger (1966) in which nuclei of gastrointestinal cells of mature frogs were transplanted in anucleate frog ovae to produce cells which developed normally through metamorphosis into adult fertile frogs. Williams (1969) has proposed that the cell types, which on becoming cancerous tend to produce ectopic hormones, contain within their nucleus certain types of DNA, the functions of which are more easily derepressed by some process, as yet unknown, which occurs during the process of carcinogenesis. While in essence this may be true, nevertheless at a different level of hierarchy of change it appears there may be a cellular basis for ectopic hormone production. This has been discussed by Weichert (1970). Briefly, he proposes that the enterochromaffin cell system derives from cells of the neuroectoderm which probably migrate into the primitive alimentary tract during embryonic development. These neuroectodermal stem cells, he proposes, are also the cells carried with the endocrine glands developing from the embryonic fore-gut which finally give rise to the functioning cells of the anterior pituitary, thyroid, parathyroid and islets of Langerhans. These cells also form the chromaffin cell system (adrenal medulla and paraganglia), the ganglia of the autonomic nervous system and the cells in the hypothalamus producing posterior pituitary hormones. Weichert develops these embryological observations into an argument which implies that ectopic hormone producing tumours and tumours in the syndrome of multiple endocrine adenomatosis arise from cells having as their embryonic precursor the primitive neuroectodermal cell and that these cells in some way retain their capacity to synthesize peptide hormones and monoamines under the autonomy of neoplastic growth. This is an attractive and unifying theory and in a qualified way is a return to the embryonal cell theory to explain some of the properties of tumour growth and function.

REFERENCES

Appleyard, T. N. and Losowsky, M. S. (1970). A pancreatic tumour with carcinoid syndrome and hypoglycaemia. *Postgrad. Med. J.* **46**, 159.

Azzopardi, J. G. and Bellan, A. R. (1965). Carcinoid syndrome and oat cell carcinoma of the bronchus. *Thorax*, **20**, 393.

Bensch, K. G., Corrin, B., Pariente, R. and Spencer, H. (1968). Oat cell carcinoma of the lung: its origin and relationship to bronchial carcinoid. *Cancer (Philad.)* **22**, 1163.

Brown, W. H. (1928). Case of pluriglandular syndrome; 'Diabetes of bearded woman'. *Lancet*, **2**, 1022.

Escovitz, W. E. and Reingold, I. M. (1961). Functioning malignant bronchial carcinoid with Cushing's syndrome and recurrent sinus arrest. *Ann. Int. Med.* **54**, 1248.

Fernex, M. (1964). Herzläscorien bei Carcinoidsyndrom und Endomyokardifibrose Pathogenetische Bedeutung der Mastzellen. *Cardiologica,* **44**, 157.

Gloor, F., Pletscher, A. and Hardmeier, T. (1964). Metastasierendes Inselzelladenom des Pancreas mit 5-hydroxytryptamin und Insulin-produktion. *Schweiz Med. Wschr.* **94**, 1476.

Gowenlock, A. H. and Platt, D. S. (1962). *The clinical chemistry of carcinoid tumours in the clinical chemistry of monoamines* (eds. H. Varley and A. H. Gowenlock), Vol 2, p. 140. Elsevier, New York.

Gowenlock, A. H., Platt, D. S., Campbell, A. C. P. and Wormsley, K. G. (1964). Oat cell carcinoma of the bronchus secreting 5-hydroxytryptophan. *Lancet,* **1**, 304.

Granlich, F. and Weithoff, E. O. (1960). Carcinoid syndrome with a report of metastasising bronchial carcinoid. *Deut. Med. Wochschr.* **85**, 1750.

Gregory, R. A., Grossman, M. I., Tracy, H. J. and Bentley, P. H. (1967). Nature of the gastric secretogogue in Zallinger-Ellison tumours. *Lancet.* **2**, 543.

Gurdon, J. B. and Uehlinger, V. (1966). 'Fertile' intestine nuclei. *Nature.* **210**, 1240.

Harrison, M. T., Ramsey, A. S., Montgomery, D. A. D., Robertson, J. H. and Welbourn, R. B. (1957). Cushing's syndrome with carcinoma of bronchus and with features suggesting carcinoid tumour. *Lancet,* **1**, 23.

Kinloch, J. D., Webb, J. N., Eccleston, D. and Zeitlin, J. (1965). Carcinoid syndrome associated with oat cell carcinoma of the bronchus. *Brit. Med. J.* **1**, 1533.

Liddle, G. W., Nicholson, W. E., Island, D. P., Orth, D. N., Abe, K. and Lowder, S. C. (1969). Clinical and laboratory studies of ectopic humoral syndromes. *Recent. Prog. Horm. Research.* **25**, 283.

Melmon, K. L., Sjoerdsma, A. and Mason, D. T. (1965). Distinctive clinical and therapeutic aspects of the syndrome associated with bronchial carcinoid tumours. *Am. J. Med.* **39**, 568.

Parish, D. J., Crawford, N. and Spencer, A. T. (1964). The secretion of 5-hydroxytryptamine by a poorly differentiated bronchial carcinoma. *Thorax,* **19**, 62.

Peart, W. S., Porter, K. A. Robertson, J. I. S., Sandler, M. and Baldock, E. (1963). Carcinoid syndrome due to pancreatic duct neoplasm secreting 5-hydroxy-tryptophan and 5-hydroxytryptamine. *Lancet,* **1**, 239.

Sagle, B. A., Lang, P. A., Green, W. O., Bosworth, W. C. and Gregory, R. (1965). Cushing's syndrome due to islet cell carcinoma of the pancreas. Report of two cases: one with elevated 5-hydroxyindole acetic acid and complicated by aspergillosis. *Ann. Int. Med.* **63**, 58.

Sandler, M., Schauer, P. J. and Watt, P. J. (1961). 5-hydroxytryptophan secreting bronchial carcinoid tumour. *Lancet,* **2**, 1067.

Schmid, M., Wenzl, H. and Uchlinger, E. (1963). β-Inselzell-Adenoma des Pankreas mit Hypoglykämie, Kambiniert mit multiplen Kartzinndtumoren des ileum. *Schweiz Med. Wschr.* **93**, 444.

Shames, J. M., Dhwandhar, N. R. and Blackard, W. G. (1968). Insulin secreting bronchial carcinoid tumour with widespread metastasis. *Am. J. Med.* **44**, 632.

Sluys, Veer J., Chonfoer, J. C., Querido, A., Hescl, R. O., Hollander, C. F. and Rijssel, C. F. (1964). Metastasising islet cell tumour of pancreas associated with hypoglycaemia and carcinoid syndrome. *Lancet,* **1**, 1416.

Strott, C. A., Nugent, C. A. and Tyler, F. H. (1968). Cushing's syndrome caused by bronchial adenomas. *Am. J. Med.* **44**, 97.

Weichert, R. F. (1970). The neural ectodermal origin of the peptide-secreting endocrine glands. *Am. J. Med.* **49**, 232.

Williams, E. D. (1969). Tumours, hormones and cellular differentiation. *Lancet,* **2**, 1108.

Williams, E. D. and Azzopardi, J. G. (1960). Tumours of the lung and the carcinoid syndrome. *Thorax,* **15**, 30.

Index